Dedication

I now know what it means when an author writes "this book would not have been possible without the help of..." I dedicate this book to my wife Ina. Without her help this book would never have been. Thank you.

Acknowledgements

The writing of this book brought together two important teachers for me.

I want to thank Dr. Bob Flaws, my first Chinese medicine teacher. He asked me if I was interested in writing a book about low back pain for lay people. He was very generous in his editorial work with this book. It is his translation of the Chinese medical research that appears in Chapter Eight. I am very appreciative for all that you have given to me.

I want to publicly acknowledge Will Evans, M.D. We worked together daily for over seven years in physical rehabilitation medicine. I will always be grateful for your trust in my work with patients, your sharing of your knowledge and wisdom, and most importantly our friendship in the Spirit.

Finally, I want to thank two friends who were willing to subject themselves to reading early versions of portions of this book and give their honest opinions. David Uher, friend extraordinaire, thanks. Nina Steinway, colleague and friend, thanks.

Low Back
PAIN

Care & Prevention with
Traditional Chinese Medicine

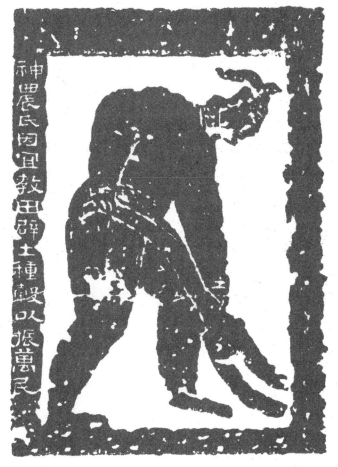

DOUGLAS FRANK

BLUE POPPY PRESS

Published by:

BLUE POPPY PRESS, INC.
1775 LINDEN AVE.
BOULDER, CO 80304

First Edition, October, 1995

ISBN 0-936185-66-X
LC 95-80458

The information in this book is given in good faith. However, the translators and the publishers cannot be held responsible for any error or omission. Nor can they be held in any way responsible for treatment given on the basis of information contained in this book. The publishers make this information available to English language readers for scholarly and research purposes only.

The publishers do not advocate nor endorse self-medication by laypersons. Chinese medicine is a professional medicine. Laypersons interested in availing themselves of the treatments described in this book should seek out a qualified professional practitioner of Chinese medicine.

COMP Designation: Original work

Printed at Johnson Printing in Boulder, CO on acid free, recycled paper with soy-based ink.

Cover design by Bob Schram, Bookends

Illustrations on pages 9, 14, and 15 by Jim Clayton with permission of William Evans, M.D.

10 9 8 7 6 5 4 3 2

Preface

Who has not had a low backache or does not know someone with a low back problem? During the writing of this book, both my wife and I each had short episodes of low back pain. It has been estimated that at any moment over 20% of the U.S. population has low back pain.

Prior to entering private practice a few years ago, I practiced acupuncture and Chinese herbal medicine for over seven years in physical rehabilitation clinics in Denver, Colorado. In those clinics, I treated people with both acute low back problems and people who had been suffering with low back pain for years. Many people were helped by my treatments and some were not. Nonetheless, in each case, I learned something from these people and am thankful that we worked together. This book is the fruit of those years' experience and education.

There are a large number of low back pain books on the market aimed at the general public. So why another low back pain book? This is the first book written for the general public that examines low back problems from both the contemporary Western *and* traditional Chinese medical points of view.

My intention in writing this book is to convey to Westerners an idea of what the holistic system of Chinese medicine has to offer in the care of the low back. This includes not only treatment for current and long-standing low back problems but also, and possibly more importantly, what Chinese medicine has to offer in order to help prevent low back problems.

To keep this book a reasonable length for the lay reader, it was necessary to make difficult decisions as to what to include and what to exclude. In an attempt to explain both modern Western and traditional Chinese medicines, I have run the risk of offending practitioners of both schools. Therefore, it is best to consider this an introduction to low back care from both the Western and Chinese medical points of view. For those who want more information about either approach, there is a suggested reading list at the end of this book.

In writing this book, I felt it important to include the Western medical approach to problems of the low back, its history, and its description of anatomy and pathology. I did this because I wanted to highlight the fundamental distinctions between these two medical systems. While these two systems can be complementary and can work together in the treatment of low back problems, their views of the person suffering from back pain are vastly different. In my experience, it is a medical system's view which determines its treatment and ultimately the outcome of that treatment.

I hope that this book gives the reader a basic understanding of how different traditional Chinese and modern Western medicines are when it comes to understanding and treating low back pain. I also hope that the reader will gain some appreciation for how a truly holistic medical system such as traditional Chinese medicine conceptualizes and addresses a person's bodily, emotional, and spiritual signs and symptoms when reducing suffering and facilitating healing.

Douglas Frank
July 1995

Contents

1
The History of Low Back Treatment in Modern Western Medicine

Spinal Surgery

The modern Western medical approach to the treatment of low back problems can be roughly divided into two periods. The first period began in 1934 with the publication of Mixter and Barr's work on surgery of the low back and lasted into the late 1950s. This period has been called "the dynasty of the disc."

Mixter and Barr were orthopedic surgeons who coined the phrase "ruptured disc." They had great success using spinal surgery to treat back pain due to the rupture of the nucleus pulposus in the vertebral disc. The publication of their work was a landmark in formulating the cause and treatment of back pain for the next 40 years. It popularized disc surgery and increased the influence of orthopedic surgeons in the care of back problems.[1]

Following World War II, there was a dramatic increase in disc surgeries. However, by the early 1950s, it became apparent that, while there were great successes in the relief of low back pain through surgery, there were also tremendous failures. As one of the early leaders in spinal surgery succinctly stated, "No operation in any field leaves more human wreckage than surgery of the spine."[2]

As the increase of back surgeries mounted during the decade of the 1950s, the number of unsuccessful surgeries grew. Statistics indicate a failure rate of between 5-50%, and a new category of back pain patients was created: failed back surgery syndrome.[3] People with failed backs tend to experience unrelenting low back pain, sciatica, and significant functional impairment. Currently each year, an estimated 25,000-50,000 new cases of failed back surgery syndrome occur in the United States alone.[4]

Rehabilitation

The second phase in the modern Western medical treatment of low back pain began in the late 1960s with the development of conservative, nonsurgical, therapeutic rehabilitation programs. The "Back School" concept started in Sweden and quickly spread to the other industrial nations.[5] The Back School approach to the treatment of low back pain combined physical rehabilitation with patient education about the anatomy and function of the back.

Multidisciplinary rehabilitation clinics that often incorporated the Back School approach grew out of the physical rehabilitation movement. Under the direction of medical physicians, these clinics brought physical therapists, occupational therapists, psychologists, massage therapists, exercise therapists, and biofeedback therapists all together under one roof.

In the early 1980s rehabilitation programs were developed for patients with chronic low back pain. These programs were designed to restore the patient to functioning rather than to eliminate pain. A combination of physical training, work simulation, behavioral modification, and education were introduced in order to attain the goal of return to functioning.

During the last 20 years, low back pain research has proliferated, as have the number of books for lay people. The major focus of this research has been the identification of pathological changes in the structures of the back and their contribution to low back pain. If you examine the back pain books available from your library or bookstore, you will see that the information in this book for the general public typically focuses on:

1. Anatomical descriptions of the low back, the spine, discs, nerves, muscles, ligaments, etc.

2. What goes wrong with these structures, *i.e.*, disc herniations, degenerative disc disease, osteoarthritis, etc.

3. Ideas about why these changes cause low back pain

4. Suggestions to help alleviate low back pain, such as exercise, diet, etc.

The Western Medical Model & Problems of the Low Back

The search for the underlying pathological changes that cause illness has been called the "doctrine of specific etiology."[6] This means looking for the origin or cause of the problem. This is the basis of the disease/illness model of modern Western medicine. The basic methodology of this model is the progression from a specific description of the disease pathology to a precise diagnosis so that a specific treatment to remedy that pathology can be administered. This methodology is based on a supposed linear relationship between pathology, treatment, and cure.

This contemporary Western medical disease/illness model is an effective one for the treatment of many health problems and is especially unsurpassed in the treatment of traumatic injuries. However, this model has significant limitations when addressing the problem of low back pain. These limitations include but are not limited to the following:

1. Even though Western physicians have the ability to describe a

wide array of back structure pathology, their ability to accurately diagnose people with back pain is only 10-15%.[7] This means that up to 85% of people with back pain do not receive a specific diagnosis for the cause of their pain. And without such a precise diagnosis, the very cornerstone of this Western medicine disease/illness model and methodology is undermined. In this methodology, precise treatment depends on a precise diagnosis. If there is no diagnosis, there can be no precise treatment.

2. It is not possible to locate *any* injured tissue in 80% of patients with low back pain.[8] Again, without a specific and precise diagnosis, it is not possible for Western physicians to prescribe a precisely targeted treatment plan.

3. The neural routes that extend from the spinal cord out into the body are exceptionally complex. This makes it difficult to locate the exact source of pain in many back problems.

4. Our current understanding of the human nervous system and how we experience pain is far from complete. "Science has only just begun a serious investigation of the mechanism of pain (or any other sensation for that matter)."[9]

5. The finding of "pathologic" changes in the tissue of the low back in people *who do not have back pain* adds further confusion to the questions of what causes pain and where in the body does it come from? In studies of normal people without back pain, 30-60% of those under the age of 35 had some degree of lumbar disc degeneration,[10] 20% under the age of 60 had herniated discs without symptoms,[11] and 24% of the people between the ages 18 and 76 had abnormal lumbar discs.[12] These findings indicate that "pathological" changes in the structures of the back may simply be a *normal* part of growing old, and the presence of such structural changes does not necessarily mean the presence of pain.

The Call for a New Approach to the Treatment of Low Back Pain

In the face of the above discrepancies between standard Western low back treatment and low back research, a growing number of Western physicians are calling for a new approach to the treatment of back pain. There is wide recognition that the modern Western medical disease/illness model is no longer adequate and effective for the diagnosis and treatment of the low back pain and disability epidemic we are currently facing.

The most recent statistics on back disability indicate that chronic low back pain is a serious problem throughout the industrialized world. A 1991 study reported that U.S. Social Security low back disability claims were increasing at *14 times* the rate of population growth.[13] An equally alarming fact is that close to 4% of the population of the industrialized world is considered disabled, temporarily or permanently, by low back pain.[14]

Many back care specialists believe the increase in cases of low back pain is due not to increased spinal disease but rather to psychological, social, and even political factors. Two back care specialists who are calling for a new approach to low back treatment are Dr. Waddell from Europe and Dr. Evans from the United States. They each incorporate psychological, social, and political factors into their models of understanding and treating people with back pain.

Waddell[15] believes that a bio-psycho-social model most accurately describes the process of back pain and disability as it is now occurring in the modern, industrial world. His model incorporates the individual's physical problem, the emotional distress that accompanies pain, and the person's social network. Waddell suggests that, rather than focusing upon pathology, the focus of low back pain treatment should be:

5

1. Keeping the patient active

2. Restoring them to function.

Evans[16] advocates that back care physicians should be teachers of health to individual patients and to the larger society. He believes education is the primary treatment of choice for low back pain. Education assists and empowers the patient to learn how to manage his or her own condition. This is in contrast to the approach of many contemporary physicians who offer patients medication first, surgery next, and education last, if at all.

Evans notes that there certainly are pathological conditions, such as cauda equina syndrome, for which surgery takes precedence over education. However, he stresses that, in the majority of cases, it is most important to help the individual realize:

1. That they have a patient-managed condition and are working together with the physician.

2. That the natural history of most low back problems is one of improvement.

3. That activity and function are of utmost importance in the recovery process.

4. That it is possible to learn how to protect the back through education and proper exercise, thus helping to prevent recurring episodes of injury and pain.

As we can see in this brief overview, modern Western medicine's focus and methods of treatment of low back pain have evolved over time. Unfortunately, while there has been a call for a new approach, the current emphasis remains on searching for the pathological changes that cause low back pain.

2
The Anatomy & Pathology
of Low Back Pain

As we have seen in the preceding chapter, understanding the causes of low back pain is not a simple task. Even the experts have difficulty making the emphatic statement, "Aha! This is what is wrong."

The information in this chapter will provide you with a basis for understanding the difference between the modern Western and traditional Chinese medical approaches to the treatment of low back pain. This is because the modern Western medical approach to the diagnosis and, therefore, treatment of low back pain is largely based on its understanding of anatomy. Thus, the first section of this chapter covers the anatomy of the low back, while the second section describes various pathological changes to these structures.

Anatomy

The spinal column

The spinal column is composed of five distinct groups of vertebrae stacked like blocks one upon the other. There are 7 cervical vertebrae in the neck, 12 thoracic vertebrae at the level of the chest to which the ribs attach, and 5 lumbar vertebrae in the lower back. Below the lumbar vertebrae lie the sacrum and the coccyx.

The spinal column is one of the principle supports of the body. Like the upright mast on a ship to which the sails are attached, the spine is the site of attachment for the soft tissues of the body, the muscles, ligaments, tendons, and fasciae or connective tissue. Unlike a mast on a sailing ship, however, the spine can move. It is the network-like combination of these soft tissues that allows the body to be upright and move in ways that we recognize as human.

The vertebrae

All the vertebrae are composed of bone and have a fairly similiar structure. The lumbar vertebrae in the lower back are the largest of the spinal column, allowing them to support the body's weight. They also have the least range of motion and are particularly unsuited for twisting.

The front of each vertebrae is cylindrically shaped and is known as the vertebral body. Behind the vertebral body is the vertebral arch with three major projections called processes. Muscles, ligaments, and fasciae attach to these three processes and to the other structures of the vertebrae so that the spine is held firmly in place yet is able to move.

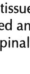

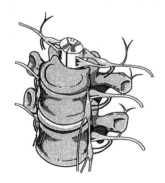

The vertebral arch also forms two small joints, called facet joints, that connect the adjoining vertebrae. The vertebral body and arch form a enclosed space, the spinal canal. The spinal cord, nerve roots, blood vessels, connective tissue, and spinal fluid are contained and protected within the spinal canal.

8

The joints of the spine

Each vertebrae is connected to the vertebrae above and below through a series of joints. One of these is the facet joint. Facet joints are important because they help the spine bear weight and prevent excessive twisting which can damage the intervertebral discs. Another important joint of the spine that lies between the vertebrae is the intervertebral disc.

Lumbar intervertebral disc

The intervertebral discs lie between each of the vertebrae. These discs form a strong joint between the vertebrae and permit the movement of the spinal column. A disc is comprised of two vastly different tissues. There is an outside ring, known as the annulus fibrosus, surrounding the inner nucleus pulposus. The annulus consists of a tissue that is both incredibly strong, like a steel-belted tire, yet able to stretch. The annulus provides a protective covering for the softer nucleus pulposus which has a gelatinous consistency.

The criss-crossing arrangement of the annulus fibers together with the gelatinous nucleus permits us to bend forward, backward, and side to side with ease. However, this fiber arrangement is easily damaged by any extensive twisting motion and thus the importance of the facet joints in guarding against twisting.

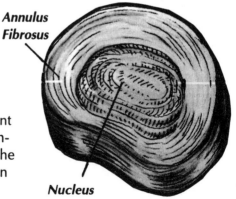

Annulus Fibrosus

Nucleus

The nucleus is the largest body tissue that does not have its own blood vessels. It receives nourishment and rids itself of waste through the process of osmosis. Osmosis is a passive process by which materials move from one area to another. This feature of the nucleus has implications for the importance of exercise as a means of maintaining the health of discs.

The nervous system

The nervous system is the body's control center and communication network. The spinal cord is the main trunk line of this system and is protected within the spinal canal by sheaths, spinal fluid, and ligaments.

The spinal cord emerges out of the brain and runs the length of the spine to the area of the first and second lumbar vertebrae. At this point, it becomes nerve roots called the cauda equina or the horses tail. This then runs through the remainder of the spinal canal.

The spinal cord is composed of bundles of nerves that run from the brain down through the spinal column and out into the body. The spinal cord connects to the nerves of the body through its nerve roots which emerge from the spinal cord and run through an opening between the vertebrae. Nerve roots often play a significant role in low back pain as we shall see below.

Once past the vertebrae, the nerve roots spread out and become the nerves that extend to all the tissues of the body. It is through the nerves that information, including the sensation of pain, is sent to the brain. Nerves that register pain are located in all the tissues and structures of the low back, making every structure and tissue a potential source of pain.

Connective tissue

Connective tissue is the most abundant tissue of the body. It protects, supports, and binds all the other tissues and structures of the body. There are many types of connective tissue. The two most important connective tissues of the low back are fasciae and ligaments.

Fasciae

Fasciae are tough, fibrous sheets of connective tissue. If you look at a raw piece of beef, the lines of tough white tissue running through it are fasciae.

The fascial tissues are an integral part of the muscular system. The technical term that is used to show this connection between muscles and its fasciae is myofascial. Myo comes from the Greek, meaning muscle. Fasciae surrounds each individual muscle cell fiber, wraps and separates the individual muscle fiber bundles, and wraps entire muscle groups.

Ligaments

Ligaments are bands of fibrous tissue that bind bones to one another or other body parts together. Most of the ligaments that bind the vertebrae together are outside the spinal canal. However, two ligaments inside the spinal canal are implicated in certain types of low back pain due to their loss of elasticity.

Muscles of the low back

The muscles of the low back are arranged in layers. The deep muscles tend to be small and difficult to reach. As the muscle layers get closer to the surface, they become larger, cover a wider surface of the back, and are easy to access. Each low back muscle performs a specific movement and has a specific stabilization function. The coordination of movement and stillness is the interplay of different muscle groups. For example, while some muscles contract to make forward bending possible, another muscle group lengthens. A healthy muscle is able to contract when engaged in activity and then lengthen and relax with good tone when the activity is completed. Chronically contracted muscles can be a source of low back pain.

Abdominal muscles & fasciae

The abdominal muscles are extremely important for the proper alignment of the pelvis and for support of the lumbar vertebrae. The abdominal muscles run from the breast bone in the chest to the pubic bone at the base of the abdomen. The abdominal muscle fasciae connect with fascial sheaths in the back which attach directly to the vertebrae of the lower back. This fasciae completes the wrap-around support from the abdominal muscle in the front to help maintain the "rigging of the mast of the sail boat" and contribute to the upright posture of the spine.

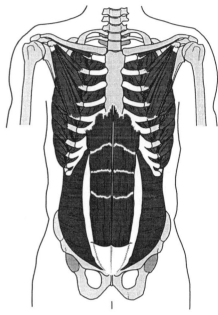

Interior Layer of Anterior Torso Muscles

Pathology

As we look at the changes in individual low back structures, we should keep in mind that they are a part of a network, a system. This means there is a dynamic and interdependent relationship between the many parts that comprise the low back. As stated above, in actual fact, pain may or may not accompany the changes of the structures of the low back described below.

Problems due to changes of the disc

The two basic problems that arise with the discs are:

1. Deterioration problems of the nucleus pulposus

2. Weakening of the annulus fibrosis, the protective covering of the disc.

Injury or deterioration of the nucleus pulposus tissue is associated with multiple structural and pathological changes of the low back. Changes to the nucleus diminish its ability to hold water. As a result, it shrinks and loses its height. This loss of the nucleus' height causes the vertebrae to rub together and places added pressure on the annulus.

When vertebrae rub against one another, the boney vertebral tissues are stressed at the points of contact. This can cause wear and tear on the vertebrae. This is called *spondylitis*. Such wear and tear can lead to the formation of abnormal boney growths known as *osteophytes*, commonly called *spurs*. This type of stress also increases the wear and tear on the joints of the spine, causing degenerative conditions like *osteoarthritis*. Further deterioration of the spine can cause *spondylolisthesis*, a condition in which a vertebrae moves forward over the vertebrae below it. This can cause pinching of the nerve roots. If a vertebrae moves backwards over the vertebrae beneath it, this is called a *retrolisthesis*.

The loss of disc height and the formation of spurs can decrease or narrow the spinal canal and passageways of the nerve roots. This narrowing, called *stenosis*, indicates that the spinal nerves and blood vessels are no longer protected from making contact with the vertebrae. Such contact can cause a condition known by various terms such as *nerve impingement, nerve entrapment, or pinched nerves.*

Stenosis can result in a number of painful conditions. One is *claudication*. This occurs with higher frequency in men over 50 who have worked at manual labor occupations. Heavy labor can cause deterioration of the vertebrae which results in spinal canal narrrowing. A primary symptom of claudication is that the person has discomfort in both legs after walking a short distance. Stopping and leaning forward tends to diminish this pain because it takes the pressure off the nerve roots and blood vessels that are compressed by the vertebrae.

Another condition that can be caused by stenosis is *arachnoiditis*. This is one of the most painful chronic low back problems. The arachnoid is one of the three protective coverings of the spinal cord and nerve roots. Arachnoiditis refers to the scarring and thickening of the sheath that covers the nerve roots. Nerve root scarring and thickening can develop through:

1. Entrapment due to spurs or stenosis causing irritation that can eventually cause scarring

2. Infections inside the spine

3. Complications from spinal surgery and diagnostic myelography that uses an oil-base material.

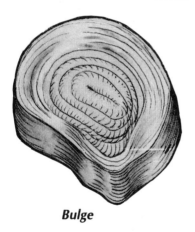

Bulge

Deterioration of the nucleus can also lead to deterioration of the annulus, causing it to weaken. This sets the stage for a critical threshold in a person's back. At this stage, excessive weight on the spine, especially if combined with twisting, can cause a bulge or a break in the weakened annulus. This is referred to as *disc herniation*. When a bulge occurs, the nucleus remains within the annulus.

When a herniation occurs, the nucleus breaks through the annulus fibers and can be thrust into the spinal canal. These tissues then reduce the space normally occupied by the nerves of the canal, creating another source of nerve impingement and inflammation.

Sciatica, inflammation of the sciatic nerve, is a common painful condition that develops this way.

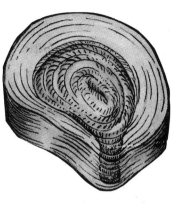

Once a disc forms a bulge or herniates, the damage is permanent. The herniated nucleus will not go back inside the annulus and the bulge will not lessen. Nonetheless, as we have seen, research indicates that many people with a bulge or disc herniation can be symptom free, or in other words, pain free.

Herniation

While sciatica is the most common consequence of a herniated disc, *cauda equina syndrome* is a more serious development. In this case, the disc material impinges upon the cauda equina nerves in the lower lumbar area resulting in a loss of bladder, bowel, or sexual function. This can be a serious condition and usually calls for immediate surgery to prevent permanent nerve damage.

The last spinal nerve problem that we will mention is the increased incidence of long-term back pain associated with the administration of *epidural anesthesia* during childbirth. This appears to be due to the irritation that develops from:

1. The material injected into the spine that "deadens" the area

2. As a result of the often awkward and stationary positions a women is placed in for prolonged periods without being able to feel that the low back tissues are being damaged.

Arthritis of the spine

Osteoarthritis is the most common form of arthritis to affect the joints of the body. It is the result of degenerative changes in the joints. Degenerative changes can occur from normal wear and tear, excessive stress on joints for a prolonged period, congenital joint abnormalities, an improperly healed injury, or old infections which damaged the joint tissues. In the spine, osteoarthritis generally affects the facet joints.

Rheumatoid arthritis is one of a number of inflammatory diseases that can affect the joints. Also referred to as RA, rheumatoid arthritis is a systemic, autoimmune disease in which the body attacks the linings of its own joints. This produces inflammation and consequently pain of the joints which are affected. RA especially affects the joints in the hands and feet. However, it can affect any joint in the body, including the spine.

Ankylosing spondylitis is a disease of the spine that causes stiffening due to inflammation of the ligaments and tendons attached to the vertebrae. Ankylosing spondylitis usually affects males in their 20s and 30s. When it occurs in women, its symptoms tend to be milder.

Ankylosing spondylitis usually begins in the sacroiliac joint and in many individuals remains there, causing low back pain. If the condition worsens, it can move up the spine causing increasing stiffness as the inflammation transforms the spinal ligaments into boney tissue. It has been estimated that mild, subclinical forms of ankylosing spondylitis which only cause some stiffness in the spine may affect as much as 2% of the population.

Problems with the facet joints

The facet joints are the two joints on the posterior or back part of the vertebrae that connect each vertebra to those above and below it. These facet joints can be affected by such degenerative changes as spurring, arthritis, and ankylosing spondylitis. The facet joints can also subluxate, lock up, or fracture.

Facet syndrome subluxation occurs when the facets become partially dislocated. In that case, the surfaces of the two facets that form the facet joint do not properly line up. This misalignment can cause irritation in the tissues and nerves in the surrounding area and thus cause pain.

The facets can also cause the back to *lock up*. When the back locks up, the person must remain bending forward. They cannot straighten up. This is because extension of the back to stand upright is too painful. Lock-up of the back can be caused by the breaking off of small pieces of the joints which then become trapped in the facet joint.

Facet fractures can occur when excessive force is placed on a facet joint through overtwisting and especially while carrying weight. Forced excessive overtwisting of the facets can cause them to give way and result in tears of the annulus fibers or disc herniation.

Sacroiliac joint

The sacroiliac (SI) joint is considered an extremely stable joint because of the powerful ligaments to the front and rear which hold it in place. In women during the later stages of pregnancy, these ligaments and others in the pelvic area soften and become more elastic to permit childbirth. Therefore, during the last trimester, the SI joint can become unstable. The joint can then become misaligned, with the possible consequence of infammation and pain.

The SI joint can also become unstable due to trauma to the pelvic area, especially to the pelvic bone in front. This can then cause pain and inflammation in the surrounding tissues.

Problems of the spine causing pain

Two metabolic diseases that can effect the spine and cause pain are osteoporosis and Paget's disease. The problem of *osteoporosis* in women is well-known. But men are also at risk for this condition. After the age of 30, both men and women have equal rates of bone loss. However, in women immediately following menopause, the rate of bone loss increases significantly. This is what makes them more vulnerable to bone fracturing at an earlier age then men. Most often, osteoporosis of the spine affects the thoracic vertebrae. Nonetheless, it can also cause the lumbar vertebrae to fracture and collapse.

Paget's disease is an imbalance between new bone formation and the removal of old bone. Normally, new bone growth and old bone breakdown occurs constantly and in a balanced manner. In the case of Paget's disease, the bones become larger, less compact, and more susceptible to deformity and fracture. When it affects the vertebrae, one of the consequences of Paget's disease is stenosis or narrowing of the spinal canal. And we have seen that such stenosis may be associated with back pain.

Problems of the soft tissue & low back pain

The main conditions that can cause pain in the muscles of the low back are strains, spasms, trigger points, fibromyalgia, and muscle imbalances.

Muscle strains develop when a muscle is forcibly stretched while it is contracted or tight. Muscle strains in the low back can occur as a result of quick movements, such as lifting or twisting, or from overdoing ordinary activities, such as gardening or mopping the floor. *Lumbosacral muscle strain* is a common problem of the low back and is most often due to chronically tight muscles. Tight muscles are more susceptible to strain when extra tension is placed on them, as often occurs when we make a sudden movement.

18

Muscle spasms are musclar contractions that are maintained indefinitely to protect or guard the body's tissues from further injury. Muscle spasms following a specific injury are due to an involuntary reflex which causes the muscles of the area to maintain contraction. Muscle spasms without a specific injury can indicate that some deeper underlying structures and tissues are irritated or damaged. It can also indicate a postural problem. Muscles can become overly active if a postural abnormality forces them to be chronically contracted.

There are some back specialists[1] who believe that muscular tension due to psychological stress is the primary source of low back pain, rather than underlying structural abnormalities. They describe a *muscle tension personality type* with similiar characteristics to what we commonly refer to as the type A personality. This refers to a person who tends to be compulsively driven to either achieve or live up to an ideal. Just as the stomach and intestines may be target organs for tension resulting in ulcers, pain in the back can also be due to nervous tension causing chronic muscular contraction.

Muscle imbalances can also be a cause of low back pain. One of the functions of the back muscles is to provide support for proper spinal alignment. There are a number of muscle groups in the low back, including the abdominal muscles, that must work together in a balanced way in order to provide this support. Thus proper balance between muscle groups is essential for maintaining proper alignment. For example, if the abdominal muscles are weak due to obesity or lack of exercise, the pelvis can tip forward. The muscle group in the back which corresponds to the abdominals therefore will tighten and cause excessive lordosis or curvature of the low back. Such a curvature is associated with increased incidence of low back pain.

Another possibility is that the *ligaments* of the low back can lose their elasticity as a result of continual overstretching or repeated trauma. These ligaments can then move into the spinal canal and

19

contribute to the problem of spinal stenosis and nerve entrapment we have discussed above.

Myofascial trigger points are specific, hyperirritable areas within a taut muscle. Trigger points are painful when pressed and produce pain that is felt in other areas of the body. This is called *referred pain*. Trigger points are believed to result from acute or chronic repetitive strain of the affected muscle. Trigger points can affect any muscle of the body, including those of the low back. Hence such trigger points may be associated with some patients' low back pain.

Fibromyalgia is a condition which has received a certain amount of publicity of late. It seems to be an increasingly popular diagnosis. In a true diagnosis of fibromyalgia, there must be generalized muscular aches and pains affecting at least three different areas of the body, and the low back is one area that is often affected. The unique feature of fibromyalgia is its association with a variety of symptoms that include fatigue, poor sleep, irritable bowel syndrome, irritable bladder, tension headaches, migraines, and painful menstruation. Women who are hard-driving and perfectionistic have been found to be disproportionately more susceptible to fibromyalgia. It is possible that this is an autoimmune disease.

Diseases of the internal organs causing low back pain

Internal organ problems can also cause low back pain. Usually, low back pain due to disease of one of internal organs is felt deep within the body and does not get worse with prolonged standing or sitting, activities that commonly tend to aggravate low back pain due to other causes. This pain tends to be accompanied by symptoms associated with the particular organ which is diseased. It is these accompanying organ symptoms which indicate that this type of back pain originates from an organ rather than the low back itself.

Damage to the blood clotting system & low back pain

Damage to the *blood clotting system* has been identified as a factor in low back pain. Research has found that there is a higher incidence of malfunction in the blood clotting system of cigarette smokers and people with chronic back pain.[2] While not all people with back pain have this malfunction, it is most notable in those with the most severe back pain due to arachnoiditis.

Summation

There is no doubt that the strength of modern Western medicine in the treatment of low back problems is its ability to actually see and describe the above abnormalities of the tissue associated with the spine. The diagnostic technology and surgical advances of this century for the first time allow the treatment of the more serious, life-threatening conditions such as spinal tumors. And the ability of surgery to relieve pain in properly chosen candidates has alleviated the suffering of many.

However, there are some notable limitations to modern Western medicine when it comes to the diagnosis, treatment, and cure of chronic low back problems. It seems that the disease/illness model which dominates and defines modern Western medicine itself may limit its efficacy when it comes to treating chronic problems of the low back.

This disease/illness model tends to focus on the structures of the back in isolation from the rest of the individual. When one views the parts of the body and their individual functions in isolation, this allows and even encourages one to act on those isolated structures in the attempt to bring about a single, also isolated, desired result– the reduction of pain through outside manipulation. It has been modern Western medicine's focus on the disc as "the cause" of low back pain that has allowed spinal surgery to achieve the prominence it has. Unfortunately, we have also witnessed in a significant number of patients the devastating consequences of such a short-sighted, linear, and non-holistic approach. Far too many patients who receive surgery for disc problems are either not cured or suffer from even more serious, debilitating, and recalcitrant pain.

The good news is that the modern Western medical approach to problems of the low back continues to evolve as it has since the early 1930s. In a search for a more complete understanding of the causes of low back pain and, therefore, more effective treatment protocols, many practitioners and sufferers of back pain are turning to traditional Chinese medicine to see what it has to offer. After all, traditional Chinese medicine is the oldest, literate, continuously practiced professional medicine in the world. This is exactly why I was hired by M.D.s to provide acupuncture and Chinese medicine at the Colorado Back School and the Center for Spine Rehabilitation. Therefore, we will now explore what 2500 years of traditional Chinese medicine can add to our modern treatment of low back pain.

3

The Basic Concepts
of Traditional Chinese Medicine

To understand how traditional Chinese medicine (TCM) treats low back pain, we first need to discuss, describe, and explain the fundamental concepts of this oldest, professionally practiced, literate, holistic medical system. As a system, TCM is very logical. Based on its theories, one can perform treatments that achieve the desired effect. Therefore, it is also pragmatic and scientific in its own way. However, TCM is a separate system from modern Western medicine, and, as such, cannot be explained by Western medical words or logic. In other words, to truly understand the how and why of TCM, one must approach it on its own terms.

In this chapter, we will present an overview of TCM. In particular, we will discuss yin and yang, qi, blood, and essence, the organ systems and channels, and the TCM causation of pain. Then, in the following two chapters, we will go on to see how TCM views the causes of low back pain specifically and how its basic principles of treatment are derived and applied.

Yin & Yang

To understand traditional Chinese medicine, one must first understand the concepts of yin and yang since these are the most basic concepts in this system. Yin and yang are the cornerstones for understanding, diagnosing, and treating the body and mind in Chinese medicine. In a sense, all the other theories and concepts of TCM are nothing other than an elaboration of yin and yang. Most people have probably already heard of yin and yang but may have only a fuzzy idea of what these terms mean.

The concepts of yin and yang can be used to describe everything that exists in the universe, including all the parts and functions of the body. Originally, yin referred to the shady side of a hill and yang to the sunny side of the hill. Since sunshine and shade are two, interdependent sides of a single reality, these two aspects of the hill are seen as part of a single whole. Other examples of yin and yang are that night exists only in relation to day and cold exists only in relation to heat. According to Chinese thought, every single thing that exists in the universe has these two aspects, a yin and a yang. Thus everything has a front and a back, a top and a bottom, a left and a right, and a beginning and an end. However, a thing is yin or yang *only in relation to its paired complement.* Nothing is in itself yin or yang.

It is the concepts of yin and yang which make TCM a holistic medicine. This is because, based on this unitary and complementary vision of reality, no body part or body function is viewed as separate or isolated from the whole person. The table below shows a partial

Yin	Yang
form	function
organs	bowels
blood	qi
inside	outside
front of body	back of body
right side	left side
lower body	upper body
cool, cold	warm, hot
stillness	activity, movement

list of yin and yang pairs as they apply to the body. However, it is important to remember that each item listed is either yin or yang only in relation to its complementary partner.

Nothing is absolutely and all by itself either yin or yang.

As we can see from the above list, it is possible to describe every aspect of the body in terms of yin and yang.

Qi & Blood

Qi (pronounced chee) and blood are the two most important complementary pairs of yin and yang within the human body. It is said that, in the world, yin and yang are water and fire, but in the human body, yin and yang are blood and qi. Qi is yang in relation to blood which is yin. Qi is often translated as energy and certainly energy is a manifestation of qi. Chinese language scholars would say, however, that qi is larger than any single type of energy described by modern Western science. Paul Unschuld, perhaps the greatest living sinologist, translates the word qi as influences. This conveys the sense that qi is what is responsible for change and movement. Thus, within TCM, qi is that which motivates all movement and transformation or change.

In TCM, qi is defined as having five specific functions:

1. Defense

It is qi which is responsible for protecting the exterior of the body from invasion by external pathogens. This qi, called defensive qi, flows through the exterior portion of the body.

2. Transformation

Qi transforms substances so that they can be utilized by the body. An example of this function is the transformation of the food we eat

25

into nutrients to nourish the body, thus producing more qi and blood.

3. Warming

Qi, being relatively yang, is inherently warm and one of the main functions of the qi is to warm the entire body, both inside and out. If this warming function of the qi is weak, cold may cause the flow of qi and blood to be congealed similar to cold's effect on water producing ice.

4. Restraint

It is qi which holds all the organs and substances in their proper place. Thus all the organs, blood, and fluids need qi to keep them from falling or leaking out of their specific pathways. If this function of qi is weak, then problems like uterine prolapse, easy bruising, or urinary incontinence may occur.

5. Transportation

Qi provides the motivating force for all transportation and movement in the body. Every aspect of the body that moves is moved by the qi. Hence the qi moves the blood and body fluids throughout the body. It moves food through the stomach and blood through the vessels.

Blood

In Chinese medicine, blood refers to the red fluid that flows through our vessels the same as in modern Western medicine, but it also has meanings and implications which are different from those in modern Western medicine. Most basically, blood is that substance which nourishes and moistens all the body tissues. Without blood, no body tissue can function properly. In addition, when blood is deficient or scanty, tissue becomes dry and withers.

Qi and blood are closely interrelated. It is said that, "Qi is the commander of the blood and blood is the mother of qi." This means that it is qi which moves the blood but that it is the blood which provides the nourishment and physical foundation for the creation and existence of the qi.

In TCM, blood provides the following functions for the body:

1. Nourishment

Blood nourishes the body. Along with qi, the blood goes to every part of the body. When the blood is insufficient, function decreases and tissue atrophies or shrinks.

2. Moistening

Blood moistens the body tissues. This includes the skin, eyes, and ligaments and tendons of the body. Thus blood insufficiency can cause drying out and consequent stiffening of various body tissues throughout the body.

3. Blood provides the material foundation for the spirit or mind.

In Chinese medicine, the mind and body are not two separate things. The spirit is nothing other than a great accumulation of qi. The blood (yin) supplies the material support and nourishment for the spirit (yang) so that it accumulates, becomes bright, and stays rooted in the body. If the blood becomes insufficient, the mind can "float," causing problems like insomnia, agitation, and unrest.

Essence

Along with qi and blood, essence is one of the three most important "energies" in the body. Essence is the most fundamental, essential material the body utilizes for its growth, maturation, and reproduction. There are two forms of this essence. We inherit essence from our parents and we also produce our own essence from the food we eat, the liquids we drink, and the air we breathe.

The essence which comes from our parents is what determines our basic constitution, strength, and vitality. We each have a finite, limited amount of this inherited essence. It is important to protect and conserve this essence because all bodily functions depend upon it, and, when it is gone, we die. Thus the depletion of essence has serious implications for our overall health and well-being. Happily, the essence derived from food and drink helps to bolster and support this inherited essence. Thus, if we eat well and do not consume more qi and blood than we create each day, then when we sleep at night, this surplus qi and more especially blood is transformed into essence.

The Organs & Bowels

In TCM, the internal organs have a wider area of function and influence than in Western medicine. Each organ has distinct responsibilities for maintaining the physical and psychological health of the individual. When thinking about the internal organs according to Chinese medicine, it is more accurate to view them as spheres of influence or a network that spreads throughout the body, rather than as a distinct and separate physical organ as described by Western science. This is why the famous German sinologist, Manfred Porkert, refers to them as orbs rather than as organs. In TCM, the relationship between the various organs and other parts of the body is made possible by the channel and network vessel system which we will discuss below.

Because the internal organs are conceived differently and perform different functions from their same named organs in modern Western medicine, they are technically referred to as the viscera and bowels. This is because, in TCM, there are five main viscera which are relatively yin and six main bowels which are relatively yang.

However, since the word viscera and especially its singular form, viscus, may sound quite strange to the layperson, we will simply use organs and bowels.

Thus the five yin organs are the heart, lungs, liver, spleen, and kidneys. The six yang bowels are the stomach, small intestine, large intestine, gallbladder, urinary bladder, and a system that TCM refers to as the triple burner. All the functions of the entire body are subsumed or described under these eleven organs. Thus TCM as a system does not have a pancreas, a pituitary gland, or the ovaries. Nonetheless, the functions of these Western organs are described under the TCM system of the five organs and six bowels.

Within this system, the five organs are the most important. These are the organs that TCM says are responsible for the creation and transformation of qi and blood and the storage of essence. For instance, the kidneys are responsible for the excretion of urine but are also responsible for hearing, the strength of the bones, sex reproduction, maturation and growth, and the low back in general.

Organ Correspondences

Organ	Tissue	Sense	Spirit	Emotion
Kidneys	bones/ head hair	hearing	will	fear
Liver	sinews	sight	ethereal soul	anger
Spleen	flesh	taste	thought	thinking/ worry
Lungs	skin/body hair	smell	corporeal soul	grief\ sadness
Heart	blood vessels	speech	spirit	joy\fright

This points out that the Chinese organs may have the same name and even some overlapping functions but yet are quite different from the organs of modern Western medicine. Each of the five TCM organs also has a corresponding tissue, sense, spirit, and emotion related to it. These are outlined in the table above.

In addition, each TCM organ or bowel possesses both a yin and a yang aspect. The yin aspect of a organ or bowel refers to its substantial nature or tangible form. Further, an organ's yin is responsible for the nurturing, cooling, and moistening of that organ or bowel. The yang aspect of the organ or bowel represents its functional activities or what it does. An organ's yang aspect is also warming. These two aspects, yin and yang, form and function, cooling and heating, when balanced create good health. However, if either yin or yang becomes too strong or too weak, the result will be disease.

In reference to low back pain the most important of the five organs of TCM are the kidneys and liver.

The kidneys

In Chinese medicine, the kidneys are considered to be the foundation of our life. Because the developing fetus looks like a large kidney and because the kidneys are the main organ for the storage of inherited essence, the kidneys are referred to as the prenatal root. Thus keeping the kidney energy strong and kidney yin and yang in relative balance is considered essential to good health and longevity. Exercises and lifestyle suggestions to develop, protect, and keep the kidney energy robust are mentioned in Chapter Seven.

The basic TCM statements of fact about the the kidneys are:

1. The kidneys are considered responsible for human reproduction, development, and maturation.

These are the same functions we used when describing the essence. This is because the essence is stored in the kidneys. Health problems related to reproduction, development, and maturation are considered to be problems of the kidney essence. Excessive sexual activity, drug use, or simple prolonged overexhaustion can all damage and consume kidney essence.

2. The kidneys are the foundation of water metabolism.

The kidneys work in coordination with the lungs and spleen to insure that water is spread properly throughout the body and that excess water is excreted as urination. Therefore, problems such as edema, excessive dryness, or excessive day or nighttime urination can indicate a weakness of kidney function.

3. The kidneys are responsible for hearing since the kidneys open through the portals of the ears.

Therefore, auditory problems such as diminished hearing and ringing in the ears can be due to kidney weakness.

5. The kidneys rule the "grasping of qi."

This means that one of the functions of the kidney energy is to pull down or absorb the breath from the lungs and root it in the lower abdomen. Certain types of asthma and chronic cough are the result of a weakness in this kidney function. Proper abdominal breathing is an important component in protecting and nourishing our kidney energy. Proper breathing is discussed further in Chapter Seven.

6. The kidneys rule the bones and marrow.

This means that problems of the bones, such as osteoporosis, degenerative disc disease, and weak legs and knees, can all reflect a kidney problem.

7. Kidney yin and yang are the foundation for the yin and yang of all the other organs and bowels and body tissues of the entire body.

This is another way of saying that the kidneys are the foundation of our life. If either kidney yin or yang is insufficient, eventually the yin or yang of the other organs will also become insufficient. The clinical implications of this will become more clear when we present low back pain case histories.

8. The kidneys house the willpower of our being.

If kidney energy is insufficient, this aspect of our human nature can be weakened. Conversely, pushing ourselves to extremes, such as long distance running or cycling, can eventually exhaust our kidneys.

9. Fear is the emotion associated with the kidneys.

This means that fear can manifest when the kidney energy is insufficient. Vice versa, constant or excessive fear can damage the kidneys and make them weak.

10. The low back is the mansion of the kidneys.

This means that, of all the areas of the body, the low back is the most closely related to the health of the kidneys. If the kidneys are weak, then there may be low back pain. It is because of this and the fact that the kidneys are associated with the bones that the kidneys are the first and most important organ in terms of the health and well-being of the low back according to Chinese medicine.

The liver

The liver is the other TCM organ frequently implicated in low back problems. Although the low back is the mansion of the kidneys and, therefore, the strength of the low back is most directly related to the kidneys, nonetheless, the liver has a strong influence on the low back due to its control over and correspondence with the tendons, ligaments, and faciae and its control over the unimpeded spreading of the qi.

The basic TCM statements of facts concerning the liver include:

1. The liver controls coursing and discharge.

Coursing and discharge refer to the uninhibited spreading of qi to every part of the body. If the liver is not able to maintain the free and smooth flow of qi throughout the body, multiple physical and emotional symptoms can develop. This function of the liver is most easily damaged by emotional causes and, in particular, by anger and frustration. For example, if the liver is stressed due to pent-up anger, the flow of liver qi can stagnate.

Liver qi stagnation can cause a wide range of health problems, including PMS, chronic digestive disturbance, depression, and low back pain. Therefore, it is essential to keep our liver qi flowing freely. One effective way to maintain a free flow of liver qi is through deep relaxation. Suggestions for achieving deep relaxation are discussed in Chapter Seven.

2. The liver stores the blood.

This means that the liver regulates the amount of blood in circulation. In particular, when the body is at rest, the blood in the extremities returns to the liver. As an extension of this, it is said in Chinese medicine that the liver is yin in form but yang in function. Thus the liver requires sufficient blood to keep it *and its associated tissues* moist and supple, cool and relaxed.

3. The liver controls the sinews.

The sinews refer mainly to the tendons and ligaments in the body.

Proper function of the tendons and ligaments depends upon the nourishment of liver blood to keep them moist and supple. Thus, low back problems involving the tendons and ligaments indicate the involvement of the liver. The connection between the liver and the tendons and ligaments is important for the treatment of chronic low back problems. As we will see below, in certain chronic conditions, both the liver and the kidneys are believed to be insufficient and need to be strengthened.

4. The liver opens into the portals of the eyes.

The eyes are the specific sense organ corresponding to the liver. Therefore, many eye problems are liver-related in TCM.

5. The emotion associated with the liver is anger.

Anger is the emotion that typically arises when the liver is diseased and especially when its qi does not flow freely. Conversely, anger damages the liver. Thus the emotions related to the stagnation of qi in the liver are frustration, anger, and rage.

The importance of the liver in terms of low back complaints is explained by two of the above facts. First, the liver governs the sinews. If liver blood is insufficient, the sinews will become dry and unable to relax. Secondly, the liver has a close relationship with the blood and blood has a close relationship with essence. Hence it is said, "The blood and essence share a common source" and "The liver and kidneys share a common source." This means that blood deficiency may lead to essence insufficiency and vice versa. It also means that liver disease eventually damages the kidneys. Thus many chronic low back problems involve both the liver and the kidneys.

We have shared perhaps more than the reader needs to know about the above two TCM organs in order to understand the TCM theory of low back pain. However, by seeing that these organs are related to numerous functions and body parts not ordinarily associated with the organs of the same name in modern Western medicine, hopefully the reader will also see the holisitic nature of Chinese medical theory. Every part and function in the body *co-responds* to other parts and functions in the body. Thus nothing stands alone to be simply cut or excised from the body as superfluous.

The Channels & Network Vessels

Each organ and bowel has a corresponding channel with which it is connected. In Chinese medicine, the inside of the body is made up of the organs and bowels. The outside of the body is composed of the sinews and bones, muscles and flesh, and skin and hair. It is the channels and network vessels which connect the inside and the outside of the body. It is through these channels and network vessels that the organs and bowels connect with their corresponding body tissues.

The channels and network vessel system is a unique feature of traditional Chinese medicine. These channels and vessels are different from the circulatory, nervous, or lymph systems. The earliest reference to these channels and vessels is in *Nei Jing (Inner Classic)*, a text written around the 2nd or 3rd century B.C.E.

The channels and vessels perform two basic functions. They are the pathways by which the qi and blood circulate through the body and between the organs and tissues. Additionally, as mentioned above, the channels connect the internal organs with the exterior part of the body. This channel and vessel system functions in the body much like the world information communication network. The channels allow the various parts of our body to cooperate and interact to maintain our lives.

This channel and network vessel system is complex. There are 12 primary channels, 6 yin and 6 yang, each with a specific pathway through the external body and connected with an internal organ (see diagram below). There are also extraordinary vessels, sinew

35

channels, channel divergences, main network vessels, and ultimately countless finer and finer network vessels permeating the entire body. All of these form a closed loop or circuit similar to but different from the Western circulatory system.

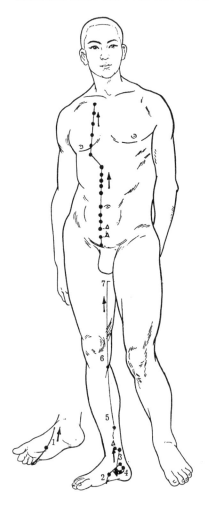

Kidney Channel

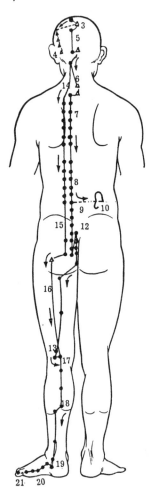

Urinary Bladder Channel

The Nature & Cause of Pain in TCM

The basic statement about pain in TCM is this:

> If there is free flow, there is no pain;
> If there is no free flow, there is pain.

This means that, as long as qi and blood flow freely and smoothly without hinderance or obstruction, there is no pain in the body. However, if, *due to any reason*, this flow of qi and blood is hindered, blocked, obstructed, or does not flow freely, then there will be pain. Thus in TCM, pain is nothing other than the felt experience of lack of free flow of the qi and blood.

Such lack of free flow of the qi and blood may be due to either of two main causes: 1) Something is hindering, blocking, or obstructing the smooth and uninhibited flow of qi and blood through the channels and vessels. 2) There is insufficient qi and blood to maintain smooth and free flow. In the first case, lack of free flow is likened to a plug of hair and soap in a drainpipe. The water from the sink cannot flow freely because something is physically obstructing the pipe. In the second case, either there is insufficient qi to push the blood or insufficient blood to fill the vessels and maintain uninterrupted flow. For instance, when a stream dries up in late summer, eventually it is reduced to pools of disconnected water. These pools just sit and no longer flow together. This is like the lack of free flow due to insufficient blood.

Besides this basic statement regarding the creation of pain in TCM, there is no other reason in TCM for the causation of pain. Therefore, *all pain no matter what its modern Western medical diagnosis* is seen in TCM as a problem with the free flow of qi and blood. Hence the TCM practitioner's job is to first diagnose the reason for the non-free flow of qi and blood and, second, to provide treatment which restores that free flow. In the next chapter, we will discuss the various reasons in TCM why the qi and blood may not flow freely through the low back.

4

The TCM Causes of
Low Back Pain

As stated in the previous chapter, pain in TCM is due to the non-free flow of qi and/or blood. When the qi and blood flow freely, there is no pain. Therefore, it is essential to keep our qi and blood full and moving freely for optimal health and well-being and especially for being pain free.

The flow of qi and blood can become inhibited in any and every area of the body: the internal organs, the muscles, the joints, and the low back. For example, when we overeat and have acute indigestion with the accompanying sensations of abdominal fullness, bloating, and distention, these symptoms are due to the stagnation of stomach qi. In this case, the stomach qi cannot move freely through the excessive amount of food and drink in the stomach. Likewise, when we bruise ourselves and blood escapes from the blood vessels and then pools, we experience a mild form of blood stagnation. In both these cases the stagnation is not serious. We feel better within a short time and are free of symptoms when the qi and blood resume their proper functioning and are flowing freely.

According to TCM, the sensations of pain due to qi stagnation or blood stasis are different. Qi stagnation causes a feeling of distention or soreness that fluctuates in intensity and location. Qi stagnation pain often occurs with strong emotional changes. Blood stasis, on the other hand, is characterized by painful swelling or stabbing, sharp pain at a specific, fixed location.

It is also possible for the qi and blood flow to become inhibited because of insufficiency of the qi, blood, or both. In this case, the pain is not severe but is enduring. If due to qi and blood insufficiency, the pain is worse after rest and better after light use. This is because during rest or immoblization there is insufficient qi and blood to keep the qi and blood moving. Movement itself helps to pump the qi and blood through the area mobilized. Therefore, movement tends to make this type of pain better.

If primarily due to qi insufficiency, then the pain is worse at the end of the day or after excessive exercise. In this case use or exercise has used up the qi and left it even more deficient. Blood insufficiency pain tends to be worse at night after it has been consumed by the activities of the day and when it returns to the liver for storage.

In the TCM diagnosis and treatment of low back pain, a practitioner must answer the following questions:

1. Is the pain due to blockage or insufficiency?

2. If due to blockage, is the pain more characteristic of qi stagnation or blood stasis?

3. What is causing this stagnation?

4. What channels or network vessels are primarily involved?

The answers to these questions directly determine what sort of treatment the patient will receive from the Chinese medical practitioner. The basic principle of treatment in Chinese medicine is to restore balance. Therefore, the *Nei Jing (Inner Classic)* says that if a disease is due to too much, it should be drained; if due to too little, it should be supplemented; if due to heat, it should be cooled; if due to cold, it should be warmed; if due to dryness, it should be moistened; and if due to dampness, it should be dried. Therefore, in TCM, two patients with the same Western medical disease may receive different TCM treatment because the cause of their disease is different. This means that every patient in TCM is given an individualized treatment based on the cause and nature of their particular pattern of disharmony.

The Causes of Low Back Pain

In Chinese medicine, there are three broad categories of causes of low back pain. These are referred to as external causes, internal causes, and independent causes. External causes refer to invasion by the six environmental excesses, while internal causes refer to damage by the seven passions or emotions. In terms of low back pain, the so-called independent causes are traumatic injury, dietary imbalance, insufficient exercise, overtaxation, undisciplined sex, and drug abuse.

External causes of low back pain

According to Chinese medicine, our qi and blood flow can be affected by invasion of energies from the external environment. These energies are wind, cold, dampness, heat, dryness, and summerheat. As mentioned above, one of the five functions of qi is to protect the body from invasion by these environmental energies. If the defensive qi is weak, environmental energy(s) can invade the body, settling into the channels, and block the flow of qi and blood in those channels. According to some Chinese doctors, such invasion by external energies can only occur if the defensive qi is deficient.

Invasion by these kinds of external energy usually involves at least two kinds of environmental energy. In other words, they do not usually invade the body singly but rather in pairs or triplets. For instance, wind often combines with heat, cold, and/or dampness. When these energies invade the upper body, we typically come down with a cold or flu. But when they invade the low back, we may get acute low back pain.

Each environmental energy has a unique set of signs, symptoms, and pain sensations that appear when they lodge in the body and cause acute low back pain. Four of the six environmental energies may cause or be involved in external invasion low back pain.

1. Wind

Wind is usually the primary environmental energy to invade the body, while the other environmental energies are typically carried by this wind. Wind refers to any unseen pathogenic factor invading the body from outside. However, it also describes the pattern of the complaint it creates. Pain due to wind comes and goes. It moves around the body just as wind moves about the earth, affecting one joint and then another. Wind blocks the qi, so the pain is achy.

2. Cold

When cold settles into the channels, the pain tends to be in a fixed location and is sharp and severe. Cold congeals the flow of blood, thus resulting in blood stasis. Pain due to cold gets worse with cold and feels better with warmth.

3. Dampness

Dampness has a fixed nature like cold. However, the pain due to dampness is a heavy, sore type of pain. It is never sharp or acute. Unlike low back pain due to wind and cold which come on quickly, dampness tends to develop slowly and have a more chronic nature. When dampness becomes lodged in the channels, changes in the weather and especially low pressure can often make the pain worse. Dampness can also involve swelling which is a sign of too much fluid accumulation.

4. Heat

Heat type pain involves redness, swelling, and hot sensations, especially of the joints. Pain due to heat can be the result of the invasion of heat directly into the body. However, in terms of rheumatic pain complaints, it is more commonly the result of long-standing dampness or cold that has transformed into heat.

Low back pain due to the invasion of environmental energies most commonly involves the combination of wind, cold, and dampness or occasionally the combination of wind, dampness, and heat. As stated previously, these energies can only invade the body if the defensive qi is weak. If there is no weakness in the kidneys or liver, then the invasion will be short-lived and the person will have an acute case of low back pain. However, if the kidneys and liver are weak, then the invading energies can settle into the low back causing chronic low back pain.

Internal causes of low back pain

In TCM, internal causes refer specifically and only to damage by the seven passions or emotions. This is not a major, primary cause of back pain. Liver depression due to stress and frustration may cause sciatica and sacroiliac pain due to the liver qi's relationship with the gallbladder channel which traverses this area. However, once back pain has been caused, emotional dis-ease may exacerbate and prolong it. Liver depression, qi stagnation will add to or aggravate any condition in the body where the free and smooth flow of the qi and blood has been affected.

It is also possible for emotional damage to create the environment in which either trauma or invasion by external environmental energies actually results in back pain. For instance, constant fear may damage the kidneys leaving the low back area weak. Thus the person may injure their back by a seemingly harmless movement. Or constant worry may damage the spleen. Since the spleen transforms the blood, spleen deficiency may result in blood insuffiency. Hence the sinews may not be nourished and may be chronically tense and tight. Or the muscles may not have sufficient qi, *i.e.*, strength, to do their job without injury.

Independent causes of low back pain

This group of disease causing agents may seem inappropriately named to Westerners. After all, isn't diet something we take in from the outside and isn't trauma something that occurs to us from the outside? The fact that diet, exercise, overtaxation, trauma, and poisoning are all considered independent causes points up the fact that, *as a system*, Chinese medicine has its own internal logic which has nothing to do with modern Western medicine nor with our ordinary use of English words.

1. Traumatic injury

The first of these independent causes of low back pain is traumatic injury. Traumatic injury to the low back is a major health problem. Trauma results in damage and even severance of the channels and network vessels. This allows the blood to flow outside its vessels and pool. Because the qi follows the blood, it also pools. This pooling of non-free flowing qi and blood results in heat, swelling, redness, and pain. The more serious the trauma, the more serious the stagnation of qi and blood.

Trauma to the low back ranges from mild to severe. Any or all the tissues comprising the low back may be involved. The least serious and easiest to heal injuries are to the muscles and tendons. The more serious injuries involve certain ligaments, the vertebral body and joints, and the disc. The most serious problem is trauma to the spinal cord.

In TCM, it is important to identify which tissues have been injured. There are specific medicinals which heal specific tissues. For instance, one would use different herbs to treat muscle trauma from those used to treat trauma to the vertebral body. However, the guiding principle for all traumatic low back injuries is to get the qi and blood flowing freely as soon as possible. It is essential to get the qi and blood moving for two reasons. First, when the qi and blood flow, there is less or no pain. Secondly, the longer the qi and blood stagnate, the more complicated the recovery becomes.

When the qi and blood stagnate in the low back, the defensive qi cannot operate effectively. When the defensive qi is not operating at full strength, wind, cold, and dampness can easily invade. If the qi and blood stagnation continues and wind, cold, and dampness have settled into the low back, the kidneys and liver will eventually be affected and begin to weaken. When the kidneys and liver weaken, the low back becomes weaker because these organs are the mainstays of its strength. As this scenario progresses, the low back becomes even more susceptible to further invasions of wind, cold, and dampness. This is how chronic low back pain develops from trauma injury according to TCM.

2. Poor diet

According to Chinese medicine, the spleen is the organ in charge of digestion. It is the spleen qi which transforms and transports the food and drink ingested. If, through overeating sweets and fatty foods, raw, chilled foods, and drinking excessive chilled beverages with meals, the spleen is damaged, it may fail to transform and transport liquids and these may accumulate to become internally generated dampness. Because dampness is yin, it tends to percolate downward in the body to lodge in the lower half of the body, including the low back. There it obstructs and hinders the flow of qi and blood. Commonly, such internally generated dampness transforms into heat and thus gives rise to damp heat mutually stagnating with the qi and blood.

According to a set of theories developed in China around the time of Genghis Khan, dampness percolating downward from the spleen can damage both the liver and the kidneys, and we have seen above how important the liver and kidneys are to the health of the low back.

Spleen deficiency with internal dampness also results in the creation of adipose tissue or fat. Fat in TCM is nothing more than accumulated dampness. This dampness not only hinders the flow of qi and blood but puts more strain on the restraining, lifting, and moving functions of the spleen qi. As the spleen becomes weak, the muscles and flesh, which are the level of tissue corresponding to the spleen, lose their tone and eventually their function. In addition, because the spleen is the root of qi and blood production, if the spleen becomes damaged due to faulty diet, this may lead to qi and blood deficiency as well.

3. Rest & activity

Rest, or literally stillness, and activity, or literally stirring, are a yin/yang complementary pair in Chinese medicine. In TCM, it is believed that too much rest damages the spleen, and we have seen above that a weak spleen may lead to muscular weakness and the generation of dampness, both of which may cause or be involved with low back pain. On the other hand, regular exercise leads to improved digestion, and good digestion leads to the creation of the acquired essence, the essence that bolsters the prenatal essence stored in the kidneys. Therefore, regular, moderate exercise indirectly helps generate essence, while lack of exercise does not.

Conversely, excessive exercise or any excessive activity, be it physical or mental/emotional, may eventually damage the kidneys. In particular, it is said in Chinese medicine that lifting objects which are beyond one's strength damages the kidneys.

46

4. Excessive sex

We have seen above that the kidney essence is associated with reproduction. In men, the seminal fluid is seen as the physical manifestation of essence and is, in fact, called *jing* or essence in Chinese. In addition, sexual desire is a function and manifestation of kidney yang, while sexual fluids, such as seminal fluid in men, are a manifestation of kidney yin. In Chinese medicine, it is believed that a healthy, moderate amount of sex helps free the flow of qi and relieves pent-up emotions. On the other hand, excessive sex can quickly deplete the qi and blood and particuarly kidney essence. Since essence declines with age, concern over too much sex causing low back pain mostly affects those over 45. However, depending upon constitutional predisposition or chronic disease, one may have to be cautious about this factor even earlier.

5. Drug abuse

Many, if not most, of the drugs which people abuse are stimulants. According to Chinese medicine, substances like cocaine, amphetamines, marijuana, LSD, and even caffiene and nicotine use up large amounts of qi in their production of a "high," "buzz," or "rush". We say that they give us energy, but that energy has to come from someplace. Where that energy comes from is the kidneys, our deepest repository of essence and qi. These drugs use this energy and eventually use it up. This then can cause signs and symptoms of kidney deficiency and essence insufficiency accompanied by low back pain.

Age

Age is not considered one of the traditional disease causes in Chinese medicine. However, after 35 years of age, our production of essence from the food we eat, liquids we drink, and air we breathe decreases. This means that after this age, we are producing less of the acquired essence and are consequently using more inherited essence. Thus it is not uncommon to encounter chronic low back pain as a symptom of aging. In particular, spinal problems such as degenerative disc disease, herniated discs, osteoporosis, osteoarthritis, chronic lumbago, vertebral fractures, chronic lumbar strain, spinal spurs, etc. are often kidney-related problems associated with aging. Therefore, the TCM treatment of these spinal problems is directed, in part, at strengthening the kidneys.

Combined causes

Weakness or other problems in the internal organs that lead to low back pain tend to develop slowly. However, it is possible and, in fact, common to have acute low back pain in conjunction with a weakness of an internal organ. For example, a person with a kidney weakness can also have an invasion of wind, cold, and/or dampness in the low back. Hence it is common to find that in any given patient with low back pain, there is a combination of causes at work, some internal, some external, and some, according to the terminology of Chinese medicine, due to neither internal nor external causes.

In describing the causes of low back pain, Chinese medicine starts from the simple premise that there is no pain if the qi and blood are flowing freely without inhibition. It then goes on to describe a number of specific causes and contributors to low back pain, all of which cause some detriment and damage to the free flow of qi and blood in the area of the low back. These range from physical trauma and diet to emotional stress and overexertion. Thus the theory of TCM about the cause of low back pain is a multifaceted one which takes into account all aspects of a person's life—physical, mental, emotional, and even sexual. This again underscores the holistic vision of Chinese medicine which cannot reduce a person's pain to a single piece of bone, muscle, or connective tissue.

5
TCM Pattern Discrimination: Describing the Whole Person

In TCM, treatment is given on the basis of the patient's pattern and not simply on the basis of their named disease. A TCM pattern takes into account all the signs and symptoms of the disease plus all the patient's other, seemingly unrelated signs and symptoms *and* the Chinese description of the cause of their condition. Therefore, *all* the person's symptoms are noteworthy, not just the one's that are specific to their major complaint. In fact, the TCM practitioner gathers so much information, the patient may not see the relevance of it all. And certainly the TCM practitioner takes much more time to ask questions about all aspects of the persons life than the typical Western M.D.

As we have seen in the previous chapter, kidney weakness can cause low back pain. However, in TCM, there are a number of different patterns of kidney weakness. There is kidney yang deficiency, kidney yin deficiency, kidney essence insufficiency, kidney qi not securing, spleen/kidney deficiency, liver/kidney deficiency, and lung/kidney deficiency. The symptoms of each of these separate patterns of kidney weakness are different although each will be accompanied by some sort of low back pain. Therefore, we need to know if a person is feeling cold or hot, dry or thirsty, if they are swollen with edema, what is the consistency of their stools, and the color and amount of their urine. By obtaining all the person's signs and symptoms, the practitioner can then begin to determine if the low back pain is due to kidney yin weakness, kidney yang weakness, or kidney essence insufficiency.

How TCM Patterns are Determined

How does a Chinese medical practitioner go about determining the pattern of illness that is causing low back pain? First, the practitioner must have a good understanding of the theories of Chinese medicine. This includes an in-depth knowledge of qi and blood, organs and bowels, channels and network vessels, and yin and yang and how these interconnect and interact. Secondly, the practitioner must understand how illness develops and how injury affects the body. Third, the patterns of illness that develop due to external invasion, internal damage, or injury must be understood and discriminated. Keeping all of this theoretical information in mind, the practitioner then obtains information from the patient.

The four examinations

Since before the time of Christ, Chinese medical practitioners have used what are called the four examinations for obtaining information about a patient's condition. These four examinations are 1) looking, 2) listening/smelling, 3) asking, and 4) palpation or touching.

1. Looking

Looking examination focuses on what the practitioner can see with their unaided eyes (except for normal corrective lens). Everything about the patient that can be observed can be useful. This includes their facial expression, the brightness of their eyes, facial complexion, bodily constitution, posture, and way of moving, inspection of the affected area, and examination of the tongue and its coating.

In particular, tongue diagnosis is a highly developed skill in Chinese medicine and a major source of information about a patient's condition. Both the tongue itself and its coating are indicators of the person's condition. For example, a thick, slimy, yellow tongue coating indicates the presence of damp heat, while a shiny, red tongue without a coating indicates a weakness of yin.

2. Listening and smelling

Listening and smelling are the second type of examination in Chinese medicine. The character in the Chinese language for this examination means both listening and smelling. The practitioner listens to the patient's breathing, the quality of their voice, or other sounds, such as a cough. For example, a person with a weak voice who coughs when active may have weak qi. Body odors and the smells of any excretions also give the practitioner useful information about the patient's pattern.

3. Questioning

Questioning the patient orally is the third method of examination. These questions include when and how the problem happened, how long it has gone on, what treatment has already been given and with what results, one's medical history in general, sensations of cold and heat, the location and quality of pain, descriptions of urination and bowel movements, sleep patterns, perspiration, headaches, dizziness, appetite, thirst, digestive disturbances, energy level, gynecological problems, and more. Because the sensation of pain due to stagnation of qi and blood differ as do the pain and aching due to the various types of external environmental energies, the patient's description of their pain is critical in determining what type of stagnation or blockage pattern exists.

4. Palpation

The last examination method is palpation or touching. Many practitioners consider this the most important of the four methods. Only by touching various areas of the body can the practitioner directly know the condition of the body and its internal organs.

The most important aspect of this method is feeling the pulse. Together with the information gained from examining the tongue, taking the pulse is central to Chinese medical diagnosis. Pulse diagnosis requires great skill and sensitivity. The pulse taken at the wrist provides information about the basic state of the person's qi and blood, yin and yang, organs and bowels, and pathogenic factors. There are 28 different standard pulse qualities described in the classical literature. For example, the pulse quality most often felt in someone in pain is classified as tight. This pulse is described as "strong and bounces from side to side like a taut rope."[1]

Thus by gathering information through the four examinations and by comparing the patient's signs and symptoms with their tongue and pulse, the patient's pattern is understood and named. The name of the pattern describes an inherent state of imbalance. For instance, kidney yin insuffiency means that kidney yin is too weak. Therefore, the next step is creating a treatment plan which will correct the imbalance implied in the name of the pattern. If there is kidney yin deficiency, the kidneys should be supplemented and yin should be nourished or enriched. Hence treatment techniques are applied to bring about this result—the return to balance and, therefore, health.

Because treatment in Chinese medicine is based on the patient's pattern as much as or even more than their disease, treatment is individual and takes into account the whole person. In Chinese medicine, it is said,

> One disease, different treatments;
> Different disease, same treatment.

This means, for example, that a patient with low back pain due to invasion by wind, cold, and dampness will receive a completely different treatment from a patient with low back pain due to kidney yin defiency. While both patients could have the identical Western medical diagnosis, each would have two totally different patterns of disharmony from the TCM point of view and each would be treated according to their pattern.

It is because TCM treatments are based upon identifying the individuals' unique pattern that Chinese medicine causes no side effects or other medically induced problems when properly prescribed. Side effects are themselves symptoms of imbalance, and Chinese medicine seeks to bring the entire person back into a pattern of balance and good health. Thus it is treatment based on pattern discrimination which allows the Chinese medical practitioner to choose just the right treatment for each individual patient.

6
The TCM Treatment of Low Back Pain: Treating the Whole Person

Chinese medicine uses a number of different modalities in its treatment of low back pain. The four major, professionally applied modalities are acupuncture, moxibustion, Chinese herbal medicine, and massage.

1. Acupuncture

Acupuncture is one of the methods developed by the Chinese to help the qi and blood flow properly. Acupuncture refers to the insertion of very fine needles into specific points along the channels. These needles stimulate the flow of the qi and blood in the channels, thereby reducing pain.

2. Moxibustion

Moxibustion is a companion method to acupuncture. Special, concentrated herbs are burned over acupuncture points and channels to produce warmth. Moxibustion is mainly used in the treatment of cold conditions to warm yang and dispel the cold.

3. Chinese herbal medicine

Chinese herbs have been described and used for over 2000 years. Each herb has a specific action on the body. For example, there are herbs to dispel wind, scatter cold, move the qi, quicken the blood, supplement the kidneys, and clear heat. Herbs are combined into formulas that address the specific pattern of symptoms the patient presents. There are a number of herbal formulas for low back pain that have been successfully used for centuries.

4. Chinese medical massage

This is called *tui na*, literally pushing and grasping, in Chinese and is different from any other type of massage offered in the West. Specific strokes have been developed to promote the flow of the qi and blood and thus reduce pain.

The above four methods can and are applied either individually or together. Many Western practitioners of Chinese medicine are trained in and practice all four. Therefore, depending on the patient's pattern and other factors, one might receive a combination of acupuncture, Chinese herbal medicine, and massage; moxibustion, Chinese herbs, and massage; or just acupuncture or Chinese herbal medicine alone. Exactly what combination of therapies are offered depend on the individual practitioner's training and clinical experience as well as personal preference.

Case Histories

One of the best ways to get a true picture of how Chinese medicine works is through case histories. Such case histories take the reader from initial examination to treatment and then to final outcome. Since Chinese medicine is a dynamic system meant to be put to pragmatic use in the real world, seeing it in action is the best and most accurate way to understand it. Therefore, below are presented a number of case histories taken from my own clinical practice while working at two physical rehabilitation clinics in Denver, Colorado. Each case history exemplifies the diagnosis and treatment of one of the major TCM patterns associated with low back pain.

Patient names have been changed and certain details have been altered to protect patient confidentiality. Each patient's main signs and symptoms are described, but we have left out their Chinese tongue and pulse signs. Tongue and pulse diagnosis are highly specialized diagnostic tools used by trained TCM practitioners. Since this book has been written specifically for lay readers, we feel that this information is too technical for the purposes of this book. Those readers who are interested in learning more about these aspects of Chinese medicine can consult the reading list at the end of the book.

One of the main purposes in sharing these case histories is to show how each person's low back pain fits into a TCM pattern which is larger than the patient's Western medical disease diagnosis.

Secondly, it is hoped that the holistic system of Chinese medicine will become apparent by presenting the most common causes of low back pain in case history format. You will see how a practitioner of Chinese medicine weaves together the theoretical information presented in the last two chapters with the signs and symptoms of a real person. You will see how a pattern is determined and a treatment plan is developed that aims at healing *all the signs and symptoms* presented by the patient, not just their major complaint. In other words, we will show how TCM treats the whole person, including their low back pain.

Along the way, we will also offer general self-help suggestions for the different types of back pain when appropriate.

Low back pain due to invasion by external environmental factors

Wind, cold, damp invasion of the channels: Jim

Jim was a 30 year old brick layer. He learned the trade from his father. He came to the office because his low back was hurting. "Yesterday I was working really hard to finish this last section of wall and was sweating up a storm. Come late afternoon, a cool wind blew in which felt good. This morning when I woke up, I couldn't move, my back had tightened up so much. And I felt this weird heaviness all over. I've been feeling cold all day and had one hell of a time getting out of bed. I just wanted to stay there."

Jim's back pain was due to invasion of the external factors of wind, cold, and dampness into the channels traversing the low back. When conditions are right, these external factors can invade the body, lodging in the channels and blocking the flow of qi and blood.

In this instance, it was late in the day and Jim was tired from working hard all day. His defensive qi that normally protects the body from environmental factors was, therefore, diminished and, at this time of day, had retreated into the core of the body, thus leaving the exterior relatively unprotected. The sudden cold wind that "felt good" met with the sweat (dampness) on his back. His cold feeling and desire to be warm indicates he was attacked by the cold. The heavy body feeling indicates the damp invasion. The quick onset indicates the presence of wind. Therefore, the TCM pattern discrimination was wind, cold, and damp invasion.

Other possible symptoms of a wind, cold, damp painful invasion include: no thirst, severe pain, swollen joints, dislike of being touched, including massage.

If the person is in good health, these symptoms will usually clear up within a day or two. However, as we shall see when describing kidney weakness, the external factors of wind, cold, and dampness can lodge in the body, causing weakening of the kidneys and chronic low back pain.

A combination of acupuncture, moxibustion, massage, and herbal medicine was used to dispel the wind, scatter the cold, and eliminate the dampness. After treatment, *all of Jim's signs and symptoms disappeared, including the low back pain.* Furthermore, the possibility of the acute symptom complex developing into a more serious, long-term condition was avoided.

Invasion of damp heat: Terri

Terri, age 26, had been feeling bad for two days. She had back pain, fever and a slight chill, an achy feeling in the body, and red, swollen knees that felt hot to the touch.

Terri's fever and chill indicate the presence of an external factor. The fever and red-hot knees indicate the presence of heat. The swollen knees indicate the presence of dampness. The body achiness with back and leg pain is due to the blockage of qi by the external factor of dampness.

Other possible symptoms of damp heat invasion include: weakness and swelling of the legs and joint pain with redness, swelling, and limited mobility.

Treatment of Terri's external invasion of dampness and heat consisted of herbs and acupuncture to clear the heat and drain the dampness.

Traumatic injury

Lumbar strain and contusion: Kim

Kim, age 36, grew up in a family that valued athletics. Prior to her job change in April, she swam or rode her bike daily and played in a women's softball league on weekends. When her job changed, Kim became very sedentary during the week and could only be active on the weekends.

"In early May, I began to notice that on Mondays my low back would be a little sore when I returned to work. But by Tuesday, the pain would be gone. Then, starting somewhere around mid-June,

59

the soreness began to last through the week. The softball games were definitely causing my back to get more sore. But the games were the only time during the week when I could have fun and play with my friends. I just couldn't give it up. I figured the pain would work its way out. By late August, I couldn't play anymore. I started taking over-the-counter pain medication because the pain was making it impossible to sleep, and it was becoming excruciating to sit at my desk at work all day. It got to the point where I couldn't sit for more than 10 minutes before the pain just would kill me."

Kim's low back pain by the time I saw her was due to lumbar strain at the chronic stage. According to Chinese medicine, the proper treatment of acute strains is important for the prevention of chronic conditions. As we saw above with "wind, cold, damp Jim," if an acute problem is not treated properly and the conditions are right, it can develop into a chronic problem.

According to Chinese medicine, acute lumbar strain is due to the traumatic severance or damage of local channels and network vessels which then results in stagnation of qi and blood. In the early days of Kim's lumbar strain, a couple of days of rest would free up the stagnant qi and blood and allow them to resume their flow through the channels. When the qi and blood flow returned to normal, the low back pain disappeared. But the repeated lumbar strain, combined with lack of movement due to prolonged sitting at work, created the conditions for the qi and blood stagnation to become more serious and long-lasting.

By the time Kim came in for treatment, her lumbar area had become weakened because the area was no longer nourished and fortified as a result of the on-going stagnation of the qi and blood. When the low back area is weakened in this way, it becomes more susceptible to the invasion of the external factors of wind, cold, and dampness. The wind, cold, and dampness settle into the channels causing further blockage of the qi and blood. This was now Kim's condition.

60

If the external factors of wind, cold, and dampness are not dispelled from the channels in the early stage of lumbar strain, then the kidneys and liver can begin to weaken. This later stage of lumbar strain is considered chronic and called kidney/liver deficiency with the presence of wind, cold, and dampness.

Kim's recovery required that the low back sinews be soothed, the channels freed, wind dispelled, cold scattered, and dampness eliminated. Acupuncture, moxibustion, Chinese herbs, and massage were used to accomplish these therapeutic objectives.

Chinese medicine has been treating sprain due to sports injury for at least 1000 years. Injuries sustained during martial arts practice created the need for techniques and medicines to help heal wounded combatants. Chinese herbal liniments that move stagnant qi and blood due to strain can be helpful in resolving acute strains before they become more complicated as they did with Kim.

Qi stagnation/blood stasis herniated disc: Tim

Tim, age 41, was a computer repairman. "It was about 3:30 on a Friday afternoon. I had just called my wife from my final job to say I'd be home in 20 minutes so we could take off for the weekend by the lake. I was lifting this computer back into place when this intense pain shot down my leg and took me down. I mean I was on the floor. I couldn't get up, it hurt so bad. That was six weeks ago and I still have so much sciatic pain that I can't get around. Nobody wants to do surgery and I don't want it either, but I don't know what to do."

Tim's primary care physician had diagnosed a herniated disc, L4-5, based upon results from an Magnetic Resonance Imaging (MRI) test. Physical therapy was not helping.

According to Chinese medicine, Tim's pain in the low back and legs was due to the stagnation of qi and blood in the governing vessel and bladder channel. The bladder channel runs alongside of the spine and down the leg, the route of Tim's sciatic pain. The governing vessel runs along the spine.

There are two stages of qi stagnation/blood stasis disc herniation. In the early stage of treatment, the focus is to get the qi and blood moving and reduce pain. Getting the qi and blood moving also helps the disc fragments to begin to reabsorb and thus reduce the inflammation that causes the sciatic pain. This can be accomplished by the use of acupuncture, moxibustion, massage, and Chinese herbs that have the function of moving the qi, quickening the blood, and dispelling stagnation due to trauma.

In the later stage of pain due to disc herniation, the focus of treatment shifts to strengthening the liver and kidneys, as well as moving the qi and quickening the blood. According to Chinese medicine, when a back problem becomes chronic, the kidneys and liver become weak. It is then essential to use techniques that both strengthen these organs and, at the same time, promote the flow of the qi and blood through the channels. It is important to note that, if the qi and blood are moved without the proper support provided by building up these organs, the kidneys and liver could be further weakened, thus making the low back pain even more difficult to heal.

Qi stagnation/blood stasis facet syndrome: Cal

Cal was 28, active, in good shape, and careful when using his back. His wife drove him to the clinic because he was bent over. "My dad had back problems and I figured if I was careful I'd avoid the problems he'd had. And so what happens? About two months ago, I was bent over playing with my daughter on the floor. When I tried to straighten up, I couldn't. It's as if my back just locked up on me. A day later, it was gone, as if it had never happened. Then it happened again yesterday, and I'm still locked up."

62

Clinical examination revealed stagnation of the qi and blood stasis with no signs or symptoms of weakness in the kidneys or liver. Cal's condition was early stage facet syndrome of the lumbar spine, the locked up low back being the key symptom. In the acute stage, the pain is due to the stagnation of the qi and blood stasis in the channels of the low back. Chinese medical massage, acupuncture, and herbs were used to free up the small bones of the back and move the qi and blood.

When small joint syndrome becomes chronic, the kidneys and liver weaken just as we have seen with other conditions of the low back. In the late stage treatment of small joint syndrome, as with disc herniation problems, it becomes necessary to use acupuncture techniques and Chinese herbal medicine to strengthen the kidneys and liver as well as to move the qi and quicken the blood through the channels of the low back.

Organ system patterns of low back pain

Kidney essence weakness: Bob

Bob looked much older than his 49 years. He'd had a rough childhood and had done his share of drugs and alcohol, which he had quit seven years ago. His low back had bothered him for the previous five years, and he had tried everything to get the pain to stop. Bob was almost completely bald and had lost a number of his teeth. His legs were weak and, as he so painfully put it, "I feel like a worn out old man."

Bob's symptom complex and low back pain was due to kidney essence insufficiency. The kidney essence is the fundamental substance of the body. The aging process is due to the gradual decline of essence. In Bob's case, the signs and symptoms of premature aging, such as baldness, loss of teeth, and weak legs, indicate his essence was prematurely weak. Because the essence is stored in the kidneys, its weakness often appears in the form of low back pain.

Other signs of essence insufficiency include: hearing loss, poor memory, weak bones as seen in osteoporosis, and sexual dysfunction problems such as impotence.

Western medical conditions that correspond to this pattern may include: rheumatoid arthritis, sciatica, chronic lumbar strain, vertebral arthrosis, vertebral spurs, and chronic lumbago.

I suggested that Bob begin to do *qi gong* practice, a sequence of specialized Chinese exercises, to help rebuild his exhausted essence. For further information about this type of exercise, see Chapter Seven. Bob also received acupuncture, Chinese herbs, and Chinese dietary recommendations. He was encouraged to eat non-steroid treated organic beef kidneys to help strengthen his essence and heal his back and related problems. It was also recommended that, for a period of time, it would be helpful to refrain from sex to further build his store of essence. This is because semen is the physical manifestation of this essence.

Kidney yin insufficiency: Shelly

Shelly was a 22 year old competitive skier. She began working out hard when she was 14 and "never took more than one day off to just do nothing." Her low back was sore, achy. It was hard for her to keep working out to get in shape for the upcoming ski season because the pain was getting worse. She awoke every night with "tremendous heat and night sweats." She always needed to be doing something. She was very thirsty and drank "at least three cups of really strong coffee a day."

This is a classic case of low back pain due to kidney yin weakness. The years of continual working out had exhausted Shelly's kidney yin energy. Yin is the substantial, cooling aspect of the body and balances the functional, warming yang of the body. When the yin is insufficient, symptoms of heat can develop, especially at night (her night sweats and heat). Since night is the yin part of the 24 hour cycle, yin weakness signs and symptoms tend to be most pronounced at night. When the kidney yin is weak, the low back tends to feel weak and sore. Because the yin is connected with body fluids, with yin weakness the person can also be thirsty.

Other symptoms of kidney yin weakness may include dizziness, tinnitus, vertigo, poor memory, deafness, heat in the chest, palms, and soles of the feet, aches in the bones, nocturnal emissions, constipation, and dark, scanty urine.

It was recommended that Shelly substitute some other type of drink for coffee because its diaphoretic and diuretic nature was consuming and exhausting her kidney yin and thus contributing to her symptoms.

Specific herbs and acupuncture points to nourish and enrich kidney yin were used. Her back pain and night sweats disappeared as the kidney yin became stronger. Shelly learned that she needed to balance her tendency of always "having to do" (yang) with resting and nurturing herself (yin).

Kidney yang insufficiency: Bill

Bill was 39 and complained of chronic low back pain. "It just feels weak and sore." When asked if he tended to feel hot or cold, he replied, "I always feel cold. It can never get too hot for me. Even during the summer, my wife will complain about how cold my feet are. I *always* wear socks to bed." Later in the evaluation, it also came out that Bill was having difficulty with his sex drive. "I just don't care about sex any more."

According to Chinese medicine, Bill's back pain was due to kidney yang weakness. The yang is the functional and warming aspect of the body. When a person feels cold all the time, it is usually due to yang weakness. Although this could also be due to weakness of some other organ's yang, such as the spleen, Bill's chronic low back pain indicated weakness of the kidneys, and his cold feet and non-existent sex drive further confirmed the diagnosis of kidney yang weakness.

Other symptoms of kidney yang weakness include: cold, weak knees, weak legs, aversion to cold, a somber, white complexion, impotence in men, infertility in women, extreme lassitude, abundant, clear urination, urination many times at night, edema of the legs, loose stools, dribbling urine, and chronic vaginal discharge.

Western medical conditions often presenting the TCM pattern of kidney yang weakness include: osteoarthritis, chronic urethritis, diabetes mellitus, chronic bronchial asthma, impotence, and infertility.

Bob was given herbs that specifically warm kidney yang. These, together with acupuncture and moxibustion, reduced his overall sense of cold and his low back pain went away. Bob was instructed to avoid cold foods and drinks because these can harm the yang.

A simple home care application that comes from Japan for weak kidney yang people is to heat a river rock (flat and round 3"X 3" and 1" thick) in a 350 F oven for 20 minutes. Wrap it securely in a bath towel so that you do not burn yourself, and place it on the lower belly between the belly button and the pubic bone. This will then give off a deep, penetrating heat that helps to warm the kidneys. (The fact that the kidneys are anatomically located above the low back under the ribs underscores that the Western medical kidneys are not the same as the Chinese medical concept which bears the same name.)

Liver/kidney weakness with cold & dampness blocking the channels: Carol

Carol was amazingly active for her age. "A woman should never reveal her age" was her motto. Her passion was hiking in the high country in search of mountain lions. She had been doing this since the mid 1930s, but lately the exertion was bothering her low back and knees more and more, "especially after hiking for about three hours." She also found that her legs were getting stiffer and that the cold, damp weather that she used to find invigorating now caused "the rheumatism in her back" to act up.

Carol's back pain was due to liver/kidney weakness with cold and dampness blocking the channels. The low back and the legs are the domain of the kidneys, so any weakness of the kidneys will show up in these areas. The knees are considered the domain of the sinews which are, in turn, controlled by the liver. Further, when the liver and kidneys are weak, it is easy for cold and dampness to invade the body and lodge in the channels.

Wind, cold, and dampness are the major external factors that enter the body to cause pain. When the kidneys and liver are weak, the defensive qi of the body also weakens, making it possible for cold and dampness to settle into the body and create chronic conditions. Together, the cold and dampness will block the qi, causing stiffness in the legs and further weakening the liver and kidneys. This causes the low back pain to worsen even more.

Other symptoms of liver/kidney weakness with cold and dampness blocking the channels are: night blindness, sensitivity to light, ringing in the ears, dizziness, aversion to cold, palpitations, insomnia, excessive dreams, premature graying of the hair, and possible numbness of the legs.

Western medical disorders that are often associated with this pattern include: osteoarthritis, rheumatoid arthritis, and sciatica.

For Carol, it was important to use acupuncture techniques and Chinese herbal medicine to strengthen her kidneys and liver, warm yang, scatter cold, eliminate dampness, and move the qi and quicken the blood. Her back and legs got stronger as her kidneys and liver were nourished and strengthened, and the pain decreased because the cold and dampness were eliminated.

Low back pain due to spleen weakness & damp heat: Betty

Betty had two health problems that were affecting her life significantly. "I'm not sure what's more troublesome and irritating, my chronic low back pain which keeps me from enjoying the theater because I can't sit still through a show, or the chronic, yellow dripping and itching from vaginitis which is taking the fun out of sex. I'm tired of taking medication for the vaginitis that comes back a week or two later. And when I take the medication, my back, which is always sore, just seems to get worse. I'm just plain fed up with the whole thing." Betty's accompanying symptoms were chronic indigestion with gas and loose, smelly stools.

Betty's low back pain, vaginitis, and related symptoms were due to the internally generated pathogenic factors of dampness and heat. "Damp heat Terri's" low back pain was due to the invasion of the external factors of dampness and heat as indicated by the presence of fever and chills. In this case, Betty's damp heat condition was due to internal factors. When the digestive system is weak, as indicated by Betty's chronic indigestion, the by-product is dampness. This dampness was evident in Betty in her *loose* stools and vaginal discharge. The heat was evident in the *smelly* stools and *yellow* vaginal discharge and itching. The qi cannot move freely through such dampness, so there is pain and inflammation.

Other symptoms of damp heat in the lower part of the body may include: burning urination, scanty, dark urination, diarrhea with pus or blood, or a burning sensation around the anus.

68

Some Western medical conditions that are usually associated with damp heat in the lower body include: rheumatoid arthritis, urinary tract infection, and ulcerative colitis.

Acupuncture and Chinese herbs that strengthen the digestion were beneficial to Betty, and thus the source of her dampness was eliminated. Acupuncture and Chinese herbs were also used to drain the dampness and clear the heat. Betty's digestion improved, her vaginitis was eliminated, and her low back pain disappeared.

Dietary suggestions for Betty were to avoid foods that produce dampness and heat, such as greasy, fried foods, sugars and sweets, dairy products in general, hot, acrid, peppery foods, and alcohol.

Liver depressive heat: Sam

Sam was in his early 40s and angry. "Sometimes I feel like a pressure cooker that just needs a bit more heat; then I explode. If someone is taking too long to write out their check at the checkout line, I come unglued. I just get so damned mad!" Sam's anger, however, was not his presenting complaint. He came for treatment of the low back pain and sciatica that was interfering with every aspect of his life.

Sam also had a tendency toward migraines, "about once a month," and pains on the sides of his ribs. "This might sound crazy, but I swear, if I get in my car and yell as loud as I can, the rib pain stops for a short while. It doesn't do anything for my back and leg pain. But, hell, one out of three ain't bad."

Sam's back pain and related symptoms are due to chronic anger and frustration causing liver depression, qi stagnation. This means that the liver losses its control over the spreading of qi smoothly to all parts of the body. This will give rise to pent-up feelings ("like a pressure cooker ready to explode") and outbursts of anger when the qi does break loose. However, because qi is yang and, therefore, inherently warm, when this qi becomes stagnant and backs up, it

69

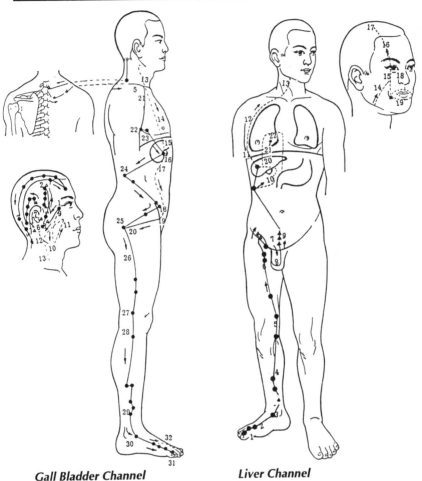

Gall Bladder Channel   *Liver Channel*

commonly transforms into what Chinese medicine calls depressive heat. This then causes pain due to stagnation and inflammation anywhere in the body associated or connected with the liver.

In Chinese medicine, the ribs are believed to be traversed by branches of the liver and its associated gallbladder channels (see illustrations above). In addition, sciatica down the outsides of the legs follows the course of the gallbladder channel in the lower body. And further, migraines in Chinese medicine are usually seen as a liver disease, where pent-up liver qi eventually accumulates to the point of venting upward to the sides of the head via the gallbladder channel or top of the head via the liver channel itself. Sam's yelling freed up the qi for a short while and brought temporary relief from the rib pain.

Other symptoms that can accompany liver depressive heat back pain can include: frequent and awful dreams and nightmares, thirst, distention in the ribs, PMS and fibrocystic breast disease in women, chilled hands when under stress, and a bitter taste in the mouth upon waking. Sciatica is the main low back pain condition associated with this pattern.

To help Sam eliminate his low back pain, it was important to get his liver qi moving because the stagnation of his liver qi was the root cause of his low back pain and sciatica. Therefore, acupuncture and Chinese herbal medicine were used to promote the flow of the liver qi and to clear the depressive heat.

In cases involving liver depression due to emotional stress and frustration, it is necessary for the person to learn to manage their emotions more skillfully. Primary self-help activities include: 1) 20 minutes a day of relaxation. This helps soothe and relax the liver qi. 2) Vigorous exercise three times a week to get the qi and blood moving. 3) Diet can be important in this type of condition. It is helpful to avoid the following foods which can aggravate liver conditions according to Chinese medicine: alcohol, greasy foods, spicy foods, and caffeine.

Blood stasis in the uterus: Martha

For the past year, Martha's low back would put her in agony whenever she had her period. "I never had any problems with menstruation or back problems until last year following the death of

71

my father. Before that, I might get a bit emotional a day or two
before my period, but now the abdominal cramping and sharp pains
in my low back are forcing me to lie down for about two days when
my period starts." Upon further questioning, Martha mentioned that
her menstrual blood contains small, purplish clots and that her pain
is relieved after she passes these clots.

According to Chinese medicine, Martha's low back and menstrual
pain are due to blood stasis. Before the death of her father, the
emotionality she experienced before her period was due to liver qi
stagnation. However, the psychological trauma of the death of her
father further stagnated her qi. Because the qi moves the blood, this
then caused the blood to become static. The sharp pains and the
clots in the menstrual blood are symptoms indicating in TCM the
presence of blood stasis.

Menstrual problems due to either qi stagnation or, as in Martha's
case, blood stasis respond well to both acupuncture and Chinese
herbal medicine. Treatment is focused on getting the qi and blood to
flow smoothly. For Martha, vigorous exercise, relaxation exercises,
and emotional support to help with her grief were also of benefit.
The exercise and relaxation moved the qi and quickened the blood,
while the emotional support she received from her bereavement
group helped her express and deal with the overwhelming emotions
which were contributing to the qi stagnation and blood stasis.

There are a number of menstrual problems that are accompanied by
low back pain. For example, "kidney yin Shelly" could very easily
develop menstrual problems such as amenorrhea, or absence of
periods, in combination with her low back pain. If Shelly's yin
weakness continued, her blood could become scant and there
would not be enough blood for a menstrual flow. Since blood is a
yin substance, if the yin is weak, the blood can also become
deficient. The occurrence of scanty blood and loss of menstruation
is alarmingly common among young female athletes.

Blood insufficiency with cold blocking the channels: Hilda

Hilda's major complaint was cold hands and feet. She had low-grade pain in the low back and occasionally her period was irregular. As a realtor, she was extremely embarrassed to shake hands with potential new clients.

A friend told her that cold hands and feet with back pain meant that she had weak kidney yang according to Chinese medicine. Her friend suggested she take some herbs for kidney yang weakness from a multilevel marketing company that sold herbal supplements, including Chinese herbs. "I figured it couldn't hurt. It was only herbs. I took the formula for a couple weeks and started to get hot flashes. This scared me and I stopped the herbs. I started to think that somehow I'd brought on menopause. Fortunately, the hot flashes stopped soon after I stopped taking the herbs. So, I still have cold hands and feet and back pain. What happened and why do I have this back pain?"

If you recall, "kidney yang Bill" had cold feet. But he also had other signs and symptoms of kidney yang weakness, such as no sex drive and the need to urinate several times a night. Hilda had no other signs or symptoms of such yang weakness. Her signs and symptoms indicated that her blood was weak and that she had cold lodged in and blocking her channels. Kidney yang herbs were harmful to Hilda because they warmed her yang and therefore further depleted her blood and yin. Thus the kidney yang herbs she took caused yang heat to accumulate within. This then suddenly appeared as hot flashes. When she stopped taking these kidney yang herbs, this buildup of extra heat subsided and along with it her hot flashes.

Western medical conditions that often present similar patterns include: Raynaud's disease, fibromyalgia, sciatica, and rheumatoid arthritis.

73

Hilda needed Chinese herbs and acupuncture to nourish her blood and dispel cold from her channels. As her blood increased, the cold was scattered. She was very pleased when her hands and feet warmed and her low back pain disappeared.

In all the above case histories, low back pain was only one of a number of signs and symptoms that the person brought into treatment. In Chinese medicine, *all* the signs and symptoms are seen as part of a *pattern*. Although the TCM practitioner focuses on the major complaint, nonetheless, they never lose sight of the forest for the trees, or in this case, the patient for the disease. Thus, in TCM, the body, mind, and spirit of the whole person are evaluated, diagnosed, and treated. This means that every patient receives an individualized treatment which takes into account the totality of their signs and symptoms. Because their entire pattern is brought back into balance and harmony, Chinese medicine heals without short or long-term side effects. This is how a TCM practitioner approaches the treatment of all health problems.

7

Helpful Hints & Self-care for the Low Back

In this chapter, we will offer suggestions about the care of the low back utilizing ideas from both traditional Chinese and modern Western medicines. These ideas are not just theories. I have witnessed their effectiveness in the many patients I have treated with low back pain, and I apply many of them in my own life.

We will begin by looking at how you can protect your low back. Then we will offer suggestions for the self-care of acute low back problems. And finally, we will provide guidelines for the self-care management of chronic low back problems.

Protecting Your Low Back

The easiest way to protect your low back is to be kind to yourself. You can do this by following a few simple guidelines. First, nurture the internal energies and substances that keep the low back strong, flexible, and upright. Second, move and use your body in such a way that the low back is well protected. And third, exercise regularly.

Nurturing the internal energies & substances

If our internal energies and substances are flourishing and healthy, then there is a good chance that our low back will also flourish and be healthy. We can start by protecting and nourishing the Chinese concept of the kidneys. This includes the kidney's yin and yang as well as the essence which is stored in the kidneys. It is important to remember that, in TCM, the kidneys reside in the lower back and that they are the foundation of all the yin and yang of the body. Thus it is essential to keep the kidneys strong if we wish to have and maintain a good, strong back.

The best way to protect the kidney essence and its yin and yang is by not overdoing. That means living a life of moderation. The kidney essence and yin and yang are most easily damaged and exhausted through the excesses of living. These substances and energies are naturally depleted through the aging process. If we overdo it, the kidneys get depleted prematurely, and this results in a wide range of health problems, including low back pain. We overdo it when we:

1. Work too much
2. Have too much emotional stress
3. Don't get enough rest
4. Engage in excessive sexual activity
5. Abuse alcohol, caffeine, or drugs
6. Exercise too much
7. Do not get enough relaxation.

If you want to immediately begin to protect your kidney essence and yin and yang, you can begin by moderating all of the above activities. For more information on the ill effects and ways to reduce the above stresses, the reader may see Bob Flaws' *Imperial Secrets of Health & Longevity.*[1]

If your kidney energies are already depleted, the best way to replenish them is Chinese herbal medicine. There are a number of herbal formulas that supplement the kidney essence and yin and yang. However, only a qualified Chinese herbalist can diagnose and accurately prescribe which formula is best suited to your specific pattern. So it is best not to self-medicate as Hilda did in the previous chapter.

For self-care, there are a number of exercises you can do that can nurture the kidney energies, whether or not they are depleted. These include proper abdominal breathing, relaxation, and *qi gong*.

Proper abdominal breathing

In Oriental medicine, it is said that proper breathing can cure 100,000 diseases. The implications of this are enormous, but simply put, it means that, if you breathe properly, there is a better chance of good health—physical, psychological, and spiritual. In Asia, proper breathing means abdominal breathing. Abdominal breathing helps to nurture the kidneys by drawing down the qi to the kidneys where it can be converted into essence and stored. Below is a simple breathing exercise from Japan which strengthens the energies of the kidneys.[2]

Find a comfortable surface on which to lie. This can be the floor or a bed. Arch your low back *only enough* so that you can slip your fingers under your back. This shows you just how much you are going to arch your back later in the exercise. Now put both your hands on your lower abdomen and leave them there during the remainder of the exercise. Let your low back come back down onto the surface you are lying on. As you inhale, allow the breath to raise the lower abdomen. It should feel as if the breath is coming all the way down into your belly and filling it so that the breath lifts your abdomen and hands. For some people this is easy. For others, abdominal breathing is difficult. If you have difficulty learning abdominal breathing, be patient and practice. It is well worth the effort.

Begin to do the breathing practice by receiving the inhalation into the lower abdomen while you arch the back to finger height. As your inhalation continues, arch the back a bit more while pushing out and up on the abdomen until it is completely filled. As you begin to exhale, count slowly to 20 and begin to lower the abdomen and back. The back should be flat when you reach the end of your count and your exhalation. At this point, before you start another inhalation, slightly raise your tailbone or coccyx to "punctuate" the exercise. Then begin again with another inhalation.

It may take some time before you can coordinate the breath and movements to the count of 20. Start easy and work up to 20. Remember, the point of this exercise is to help strengthen the lower abdomen, not to frustrate yourself.

Relaxation

The second way we nurture and protect the kidney energy is through deep relaxation. Every movement we make, every thought we think, and every feeling we feel consumes some qi, blood, and essence. By overdoing, we excessively consume qi, blood, and essence and thus weaken our kidneys, the root of the body according to Chinese medicine. In addition, when our kidneys become weak, they usually first become kidney yin deficient before going on to become both yin and yang deficient. It is said in Chinese medicine that, "Excesses of the seven emotions transform into fire." And fire which is yang consumes and exhausts yin. Therefore, deep relaxation achieves two ends. First, it calms and slows all the body's functions and thus its expenditure of qi, blood, and essence. Secondly, it calms the spirit or mind and helps clear fire due to emotional stress. Thus yin is conserved and protected from damage.

In order for deep relaxation to benefit our body and mind, the relaxation technique used must include these three principles:

1. Allowing the breath to come into the lower abdomen

2. Allowing the mind to be focused upon something other than thoughts and feelings

3. Allowing the body to be physically at ease.

There are a number of ways to practice relaxation which achieve these three basic goals. However, one convenient way is to use a relaxation tape. If you use a relaxation tape, pay particular attention to allowing the breath to come into the lower abdomen.

I have developed a simple relaxation technique that is based upon mindfulness meditation for my patients. It is called GAB (Gravity, Awareness & Breath). Lie down and get comfortable. Place your hands on your belly. Give yourself over to gravity. Allow what you are lying on to hold you. Surrender to it. Allow the breath to come into your belly. Put your awareness, your attention, on the breath entering and leaving your belly. Feel your hands rise and fall with the breath. When you find yourself thinking about anything, gently bring your awareness back to the breath going in and out of your belly.

Doing a daily 20 minute relaxation practice will have a cumulative effect over time on the mind and body. It is said in China of this type of practice, "Small results in 100 days; big results in 1000." By small results, the Chinese mean beneficial changes in blood pressure, sleep, appetite, elimination, mood, energy, and the warmth in one's hands and feet. By large results, they mean changing the way we relate to stressful situations. In either case by creating a "psychic oasis" daily and allowing the breath to move in and out of the lower abdomen, we help the qi flow normally throughout the body, we help the qi accumulate as essence to be stored in the kidneys, we calm our spirit, and we slow the consumption of qi, blood, and essence.

A healthy diet

As we have already seen, a healthy diet is important for the creation of sufficient qi, blood, and essence. In particular, it is important to keep our spleens strong. Throughout most of this book, we have emphasized the role of the liver and kidneys in the health and well-being of the low back. However, preventively, the spleen is also

79

extremely important. In Chinese medicine, the spleen governs digestion and the manufacture of qi and blood from the products of digestion.

If, through faulty diet or what the Chinese call an unregulated or undisciplined diet, we eat too much sweet and fats, drink too many cold liquids with meals, or simply overeat, this may damage the spleen. Once the spleen is damaged, it may not produce sufficient qi and blood on the one hand but may generate pathological dampness on the other. Sufficient fresh qi and blood is necessary to nourish the blood and fill the essence and, therefore, indirectly for the health of the liver and kidneys. While dampness may obstruct and hinder the free flow of qi and blood through the low back.

Therefore, a proper diet is one of the essential parts of any program for protecting the low back and promoting its health. For more information on Chinese medicine and a healthy diet, the reader may see Bob Flaws' *Arisal of the Clear: A Simple Guide to Healthy Eating According to Traditional Chinese Medicine.*[3]

Qi gong

One of the oldest systems of exercise for correcting health problems and developing energy, including essence, comes from China under the name of *qi gong.* Literally, *qi gong* means qi work, and there are specific *qi gong* exercises for every type of health problem, including pain in the low back. Many TV documentaries on China show people in the public gardens practicing *qi gong* in the morning. *Qi gong* practice is designed to coordinate the mind, the breath, and physical movement. Thus the qi and blood flow harmoniously through the channels, the spirit is calmed, and pain relieved. It is best to receive instructions for *qi gong* exercises from a qualified teacher, but if that is not possible, there are books and video tapes to learn from. See the suggested reading list for further information on such instructional aides.

One simple *qi gong* exercise is to sit comfortably in a chair with your back straight. Allow the breath to come into your abdomen and your body to relax. As the breath comes into the body, imagine the breath coming up your back and over the top of your head. Then imagine the breath coming down the front of your body as you exhale. With each inhalation, visualize and try to feel the breath traveling up the back over the spine, and with each exhalation visualize and try to feel the breath traveling down the center of the front of the body. Thus the breath forms a wheel revolving ceaselessly with each cycle of respiration. Let your mind relax and don't force anything. Just receive the breath and let it go up the back and down the front, up the back and down the front. *Qi gong* practitioners call this the small microcosmic circuit.

Moving properly with good body mechanics

The second way to protect your back is to move properly. The term for this in Western culture is good body mechanics. In TCM terms, proper movement originates from the lower abdomen. In Chinese, this is called the lower *dan tian*. This means the lower field of elixir and refers to the place kidney essence is stored in the body. This area of the lower abdomen also happens to be the body's physical center of gravity.

It is fairly common knowledge that it is best to use the legs instead of the back when lifting an object, and it is also best to hold the object as close to the body as possible when lifting. But, as with many good suggestions, we tend to ignore or forget when we are in a hurry. To save time, we do without paying attention to *how* we are doing. When we are in a hurry, we tend to be off-balance and "fall back" on our backs to do the work. This kind of movement puts the back at greater risk for injury since it is physically not designed to function in this way.

The following three movement principles help people learn how to protect the low back, whether or not there is a low back problem:

1) you can only protect your back in the present moment; 2) move from your center of gravity; and 3) be balanced in all activity.

1. You can only protect your back in the present moment

You can only protect your back in the present moment means being present and aware of what you are doing moment-by-moment throughout your daily activities. By synchronizing mind and body, we come back into the present moment and do not drift off into daydreams.

It does no good to say to yourself when you wake up in the morning, "I'm going to protect my back today," and then jump out of bed using poor body mechanics. The basis for all good body movement, body mechanics, begins with awareness of how one moves.

2. Move from your center of gravity

Moving from your center of gravity means moving from below your belly button. The best protection for the low back is to keep your center of gravity squarely over your feet in all activity. When we move in this way throughout our day, we are balanced.

3. Be balanced in all activity

Being balanced in all activity is best explained by a series of experiments. Pay attention to whether you are centered in your activities today. Do you reach for things rather than move in close and establish stability before lifting? When you rise up from a chair, do you lean forward, or do you move to the front of the chair and allow your legs to lift you out of the chair? When you put on your clothes, do you stand wobbling on one leg or do you sit down? If someone was to say "stop" while you were in the middle of an activity, could you hold that posture comfortably without needing to shift your weight to get balanced?

82

One of the best methods for learning how to move in a balanced way is the practice of *tai ji quan*, also written in the West, *T'ai Chi Ch'uan*. This is a movement practice developed hundreds of years ago in China. The practice of *tai ji quan* teaches a person how to be aware and move from their center in all daily activity. *Tai ji quan* is a sequence of linked movements done in slow, mindful motion. The most popular form in the West takes about 15 minutes to practice. It is best to learn *tai ji quan* from a qualified instructor. However, if that is not possible, there are excellent instructional video tapes available that demonstrate the practice. For information about *tai ji quan* tapes, see the suggested reading list in the back of this book.

Exercise regularly to keep your body healthy

The third suggestion for protecting and supporting your low back is to exercise regularly. This means aerobic type workouts 3-4 times a week for 20-30 minutes each time. An aerobic workout is one which raises your heart rate 80% above normal and keeps it elevated for as long as the exercise continues. Since most peoples' heart rate is around 75 beats per minute, this means raising your heart rate to 125 beats per minute.

According to Chinese medicine, exercise promotes the free and normal flow of qi and blood. It releases any pent-up qi and quickens the blood, thus dispelling stasis. It also stimulates the digestion and the production of fresh qi and blood. In terms of Western medicine, beside the benefits to your cardiovascular system and the sense of well-being that comes with being in shape, there are some specific benefits for the low back.

Disc health

In order to maintain healthy discs, there must be a good flow of fluids through the area. The intervertebral discs do not come directly in contact with any blood vessels. Remember, they get their nutrition through the process of osmosis. This means that the cells that comprise the disc only get the nutrients they need if the fluids that bathe them move. Exercise is the best and only real way of assisting this process of osmosis and keeping the discs well-nourished.

Abdominal muscles

The abdominal muscles are a part of the wrap-around support for the low back. If these muscles become weak due to poor overall conditioning or obesity, the proper support for the lumbar spine will be lacking. For a healthy back, it is, therefore, important to keep your abdominal muscles well-toned and to maintain proper body weight. One form of exercise that can be especially helpful to both the abdominal muscles and the low back is Pilates work. This form of exercise combines both Eastern type movements with Western physical therapy practices to stretch, strengthen, and tone the muscles of the back and abdomen.

Acute Low Back Problems

Points to remember when you have acute low back pain

Acute low back problems are defined as "activity intolerance due to low back, or back-related leg pains of less than three months duration."[4] Therefore, if your low back has just started hurting or has been hurting for a short while, keep in mind that 90% of all acute low back pain problems naturally get better within ten to twelve weeks *without medical intervention.*[5]

However, even though we may know that 90% of all back pain gets better, we may, nonetheless, worry that we are in the 10% that won't improve. It is difficult enough to be in pain. It is more difficult to be in pain and wondering if there is something seriously wrong with your back. This is especially true if the pain is intense and has lasted for more than a few days. Therefore, it is important to do your best to anchor yourself on the sure ground of factual information,

84

rather than succumbing to the fears that arise in the face of uncertainty.

Questions to ask yourself when you have acute low back pain

If your low back is hurting due to either a specific incident or for unknown reasons, ask yourself the following questions:

1. Have I developed any other health problems recently? Have you developed a fever or chills, unexplained weight loss, or do you have a history of cancer?

2. Have my bowel and bladder functions changed?

3. Have my legs lost their strength?

If the answer to any of the above questions is yes, you should see a doctor immediately. Acute low back pain accompanied by any one of the above symptoms should receive immediate medical assessment.

If you answered no to these three questions, your back will most likely get better within the next few months. But, even so, most of us like to do something to help our recovery along. Traditional Chinese Medicine is an effective approach to resolving low back problems. Healing time can be reduced and pain can be managed through the use of acupuncture, moxibustion, Chinese herbal medicines, and massage.

What to do if your physician wants to do tests of your back

If you do consult a Western medical doctor, it is best to seek the advice from a doctor who is wise about back problems and who emphasizes conservative treatment. This means an approach similiar to the one described by Drs. Waddell and Evans in Chapter One. However, if the doctor you see wants to do tests of your back, consider these facts:

1. No findings of degenerative structural changes by *any* imaging techniques can reliably predict the course of your recovery.[6] Many people have pathological changes without symptoms of pain. Diagnostic techniques can show what is physically wrong with your back, but they cannot guarantee that the identified change is the cause of your pain. Neither can test results tell how long your pain will last.

2. No structural changes alter the choices of conservative treatment modalities.[6] Regardless of the structural changes that are found in your back, the basic Western medical approach to treatment is going to be the same.

3. No surgical procedure can meaningfully alter your rate of improvement by altering the structure of your back.[6] If a physician recommends spinal surgery, it is wise to seek a second opinion. Make certain that both physicians arrive at the same diagnosis before you agree to undergo spinal surgery. The most successful results from spinal surgery occur in patients who have received an *accurate* diagnosis of a problem requiring surgery.

4. In the long term, there is little or no difference between low back pain groups who underwent surgery and those who were treated more conservatively without surgery. This includes people with sciatic pain due to disc surgery.[7]

5. Before submitting to a myelogram, it is important to know that myelograms with an oil-based medium have been found to cause high incidences of arachnoiditis.[8] There are also reports of patients who have received myelograms with a water-soluble medium who have subsequently been rendered paraplegic.[9]

The importance of keeping active with acute low back pain

The most common error people make in self-care for acute low back pain is too much bed rest. Research on acute low back pain shows that keeping active within one's limits is important for recovery from acute low back pain. A study published in *The New England Journal of Medicine* compared the recovery rates of two groups with acute low back pain.[10] One group got complete bed rest for two days with back-mobilization exercises, while the other group continued with their ordinary daily activities as tolerated. The results of this study indicated that the best recovery rates were found in the group that maintained a normal activity level.

It is important to note that most back care specialists recommend no more than two days of complete bed rest and only if absolutely necessary. More than four days of bed rest may have potentially debilitating effects.[11] Prolonged bed rest causes the body to decondition, and there is no proven therapeutic benefit to longer bed rest. It is important to be up and moving within one's limits. This is the Goldilocks approach: "Not too much and not too little!"

Medication

The safest medications for pain with the least amount of possible side effects are Chinese herbal formulas. Chinese herbs in combination with acupuncture can be an effective approach for most acute low back pain problems. If you decide to take Western medication for acute low back pain acetaminophen is recommended as being safest.

Nonsteroidal anti-inflammatory drugs (NSAIDs), including aspirin and ibuprofen are effective in reducing pain.[12] Unfortunately, they can also cause gastrointestinal irritation and even ulceration or, less commonly, renal or allergic problems. Muscle relaxants seem to be no more effective than NSAIDs. Muscle relaxant side effects can include drowsiness in up to 30% of patients. Opioids also appear no more effective than the above mentioned analgesics for low back symptoms. The risks of opioid use include drowsiness, decreased reaction time, clouded judgment, possible misuse, and drug dependence.

It is important to note that the long-term use of acetaminophen and NSAIDs is controversial. Research has found that taking more than 1000 acetaminophen pills in a lifetime doubles the likelihood of kidney disease. And taking more than 5000 NSAID pills other than aspirin also increases the incidence of kidney disease.[13] These medications are very impactful to the entire body. If these medications are taken they should be used only for the short term management of acute pain conditions and not for the ongoing daily management of chronic pain.

Epidurals

Some women experience intense low back pain during labor for which they receive epidural injections of nerve blocking medication. However, there are risks to the low back when receiving epidural injections. One study of women who received epidurals during childbirth concluded that 8% will experience long-term backache.[14]

Chronic Low Back Pain

There are no easy solutions to the management of chronic or enduring low back pain. Nonetheless, the following principles and ideas derived from Oriental medicine theory and clinical experience have been helpful for many longterm low back pain sufferers.

Get your qi & blood moving

Because pain is due to the non-free flow of qi and blood, according to TCM, it is vital to get the qi and blood moving. The following are ways to get your qi and blood flowing freely and properly.

Chinese medicine

Chinese medicine, including acupuncture, moxibustion, Chinese herbal medicine, and Chinese medical massage, are particularly effective for the treatment of chronic low back problems. The optimal treatment for such chronic conditions is two-fold. First, the internal organs, especially the liver and kidneys, need to be strengthened. This is best accomplished by Chinese herbal medicines taken internally. Secondly, the qi and blood need to be moved. This can be accomplished through the use of acupuncture, moxibustion, massage, Chinese herbs applied to the affected area, and self-care exercises such as *qi gong*, abdominal breathing, and deep relaxation.

For patients with chronic low back pain, I highly recommend Chinese medicine, including acupuncture and moxibustion. I would not have been retained by the Colorado Back School and the Center for Spine Rehabilitation for over 7 years if Chinese medicine was not an effective treatment for low back pain. In Chapter Eight we have included abstracts of a number of recent Chinese research reports showing the effectiveness of Chinese medicine for the treatment of acute and chronic low back pain.

Exercise

The easiest and least expensive way to move the qi and quicken the blood is exercise. Two basic forms of exercise are best suited for low back problems. The first is *qi gong*-type exercises as described above. These types of exercises are contemplative and work simultaneously with the mind and body. The second is aerobic

89

exercises, such as swimming, quick walking, and biking. If you are "out of shape," you should get a physical examination before beginning strenuous exercise.

Vigorous exercise has all the benefits with which we are all familiar *plus an added benefit for people with low back pain.* There is a relationship between certain low back pain problems and dysfunction of the blood clotting system. For these individuals, blood clots form but do not clear away as they should. From a TCM point of view, this is considered a blood stagnation problem. Vigorous exercise helps activate the blood clotting system to work properly and thereby reduce this type of low back pain. Exercise alone may not stop the low back pain, but it definitely contributes significantly to further healing and reduction of pain.

Working with one's emotions

There are times when a doctor may tell a patient that there is no further medical intervention available for alleviating their chronic pain. The patient is told that they will "just have to learn to live with it." This is like throwing someone into the deep end of a pool without giving them swimming lessons. Like everything in life that is difficult, there are techniques which make coping easier.

It is a challenge to live with the thoughts and feelings that accompany chronic physical pain. It is easy to slip into depression and hopelessness in the face of a future filled with unending pain. Chronic pain places an enormous stress on the person, a marriage, family life, and one's ability to work.

An excellent book for learning how to deal with physical pain and its accompanying emotional/spiritual effects is *Full Catastrophe Living* by Jon Kabat-Zinn.[15] This book is based upon Kabat-Zinn's successful pain management program which includes teaching mindfulness meditation to chronic pain patients. I highly recommend this book and its companion audiotapes if you experience chronic pain or if you want to learn the practical benefits of meditation.

It is my personal and professional clinical experience over more than a decade in treating patients with chronic, debilitating low back pain that relaxation tapes, biofeedback training, self-hypnosis, or any other discipline that promotes body/mind synchronization can help with chronic pain.

Creativity

Family members and friends can only listen to reports about pain for so long before they don't want to hear about it any more. This poses a difficulty to the person in pain because there is a natural need to express one's experience, especially the experience of ongoing pain.

We must remember that the human mind is creative. If you watch a young child at play, you see how her mind continuously creates one playful world after another. As adults, we can see the creative nature of the mind in the endless daydreams that our own minds create. Unfortunately, when we are in chronic pain, our thoughts tend toward creating an inner world that is filled with a great deal of suffering.

We are much kinder to ourselves when we directly and consciously work with the fundamentally creative nature of the mind. When we give creative expression to our experience of pain, we can enrich our lives, rather than being victimized by what our mind creates.

Many people say, "I'm not creative" or "I don't know how." When we were young, we needed no experience or special talent to paint, draw, or play. If playing with the fundamental creative nature of the mind brings such delight to children, why not allow yourself the same enjoyment? You can see what it is like to play, create, and give full expression to what is going on in the life you inhabit, including the pain. Is there something that you used to like to do that you have not done for years? Painting, dancing, singing, stand-up comedy?

Those who have something better to do suffer less

The painful sensations in our body ebb and flow. When our attention is continuously focused on the sensation of pain and ridding ourselves of those sensations, our world becomes very small. Our pain becomes the center of the universe with everything revolving around it.

If there is a larger vision and purpose to our life, our suffering is included in that larger field. The sensations of pain may be present, but they are balanced within the larger scope of what we want to accomplish in life. If we have a meaningful mission or goal, the physical sensations of our body may be unpleasant, but they will not stop us from living a full and productive life.

8
Recent Research on Chinese Medical Treatment of Low Back Pain

Acupuncture and Chinese medicine are relatively recent arrivals to the West. Some readers may be skeptical about the benefits of acupuncture and Chinese medicine. Indeed, recent research performed and published in the West has suggested that acupuncture is not as effective as other treatment modalities for low back pain. These results simply do not match with my clinical experience in treating low back pain or the research that comes from China. Volumes of research done in China, the place where acupuncture was created and has flourished for more than 2000 years, clearly demonstrates that acupuncture and its adjunctive therapies can indeed successfully treat both acute and chronic low back pain, including sciatica.

The research below supports the use of acupuncture for low back pain. It is only a random sampling of Chinese research on the acupuncture treatment of low back pain published in China in 1993-94. Because the majority of Western researchers do not have access to such information published only in Chinese, it is possible for a single study published in English to present an erroneous and inaccurate point of view. The following research is presented as a counterbalance to recent inaccurate accounts that acupuncture cannot help heal the causes of low back pain.

Acute lumbar sprain

Wang Wen-yuan *et al.*, in *Bei Jing Zhong Yi (Beijing Chinese Medicine)*, #1, 1993, reported on 5461 cases of neck, shoulder, low back, and knee pain using acupuncture. Of these, more than 4000 cases, 215 suffered from acute lumbar sprain and 186 from sciatic pain. Their ages ranged between 29-85 years old, and there were 55.3% men and 44.6% women in this study. Patients received acupuncture 1 time per day for a total of 10 treatments. Of the total 5461 cases so treated, 76.10% were cured and the total improvement rate was 97.2%.

Shu Hong-wen, in *Shang Hai Zhen Jiu Za Zhi (Shanghai Journal of Acupuncture & Moxibustion)*, #3, 1994, reported on the treatment of 129 cases of acute lumbar sprain by needling a single point. The ages of these patients ranged from 19-82 years old, with 43 years of age being the average. They had suffered from 2 hours to 15 days, with an average duration of pain for 3 days. The patients who received acupuncture at this single point were compared with a control group who received acupuncture at a group of somewhat more standard points. In the single point group, there were 114 cures for a cure rate of 88%. The remaining 15 patients all showed marked improvement. Of those, 73 were cured *in a single treatment,* 33 in 2 treatments, and 8 in 3 treatments. In the control group, 60% were cured, 17% were markedly improved, and 23% showed fair improvement. *This means that all the cases in both groups improved after receiving acupuncture treatment.*

Kang Jin-qi *et al.*, in *Shang Hai Zhen Jiu Za Zhi (Shanghai Journal of Acupuncture & Moxibustion)*, #4, 1994, also reported on the acupuncture treatment of acute low back sprain. They treated 130 cases who had been suffering from 1/2-7 days. One hundred four patients were men and 26 were women. Their ages ranged from 27-82 years. Of these 130 cases, 110 or 85% were cured *with 1 treatment,* while 20 or 15% were cured with 2 treatments. Only 6

94

cases out of 130 were not cured in either 1 or 2 acupuncture treatments.

Degenerative disc disease

Guo Jian-hua, in *Jiang Su Zhong Yi (Jiangsu Chinese Medicine)*, #4, 1994, reported that, in treating 78 cases with prolapsed intervertebral discs with a combination of acupuncture, massage, heat lamps, and acupressure, 56 cases or 2% were cured, 15 cases or 19.2% were markedly improved, 5 cases or 6% showed fair improvement, and only 2 cases or 2.8% got no result. This is a total improvement rate of 97.2%.

Wu Shi-qian, in *Tian Jin Zhong Yi (Tianjin Chinese Medicine)*, #4, 1994, reported on 50 cases of lumbar disc protrusion treated with acupuncture. Of these 50 patients, 30 were men and 20 were women. Their ages ranged from 30-60 years. They received acupuncture at 4-6 points per treatment, and 1 treatment every day for 10 days equaled 1 course of therapy. Typically, patients received 3 full courses of therapy. Of these 50 cases, 40 cases or 80% were cured, 8 experienced marked improvement, and 2 got no results. Thus the total improvement rate in this study was 96%.

These studies demonstrate that treatment by qualified and experienced acupuncturists can relieve both acute and chronic low back pain. Western researchers may argue that these studies were not "scientific studies" with a control group and experimental group. These type of empirical studies cannot be done with acupuncture. The studies cited here took place in clinics with real low back pain patients of all ages and both sexes. *In all these studies*, the cure rate was above 60% and the total improvement rate was above 95%.

In the West, most acupuncturists use a combination of acupuncture, massage, Chinese herbal medicine, Chinese dietary therapy, and various types of Chinese exercise therapy. The modern Chinese medical literature shows that *any one of these modalities* can cure or significantly improve low back pain. For instance, Qiu Wang-xing, in *Zhe Jiang Zhong Yi Za Zhi (Zhejiang Journal of Chinese Medicine)*, #12, 1993, reported on the treatment of 20 cases of acute lumbar sprain with a formula first recorded in the Chinese medical literature around 200 C.E. Of these 20 cases, 6 were cured in 3 days and 14 were cured in 4-6 days. However, it is my experience that even better results are achieved, especially for chronic low back pain, when these modalities are used together as they are by the majority of Western practitioners of acupuncture and TCM.

9

Finding a Professional Practitioner of Traditonal Chinese Medicine

Traditional Chinese medicine is one of the fastest growing holistic health care systems in the West. At the present time, there are 50 colleges in the United States alone which offer 3-4 year training programs in acupuncture, moxibustion, Chinese herbal medicine, and Chinese medical massage. In addition, many of the graduates of these programs have done postgraduate studies at colleges and hospitals in China, Taiwan, Hong Kong, and Japan. Further, a growing number of trained Oriental medical practitioners have immigrated from China, Japan, and Korea to practice acupuncture and Chinese herbal medicine in the West.

Traditional Chinese medicine, including acupuncture, is a discreet and independent health care profession. It is not simply a technique that can easily be added to the array of techniques of some other health care profession. The study of Chinese medicine, acupuncture, and Chinese herbs is as rigorous as is the study of allopathic, chiropractic, naturopathic, or homeopathic medicine. Previous training in any one of these other systems does not automatically confer competence or knowledge in Chinese medicine. In order to get the full benefits and safety of Chinese medicine, one should seek out professionally trained and credentialed practitioners.

In the United States, recognition that acupuncture and Chinese medicine are their own independent professions has led to the creation of the National Commission for the Certification of Acupuncturists (NCCA). This commission has created and administers a national board examination in both acupuncture and Chinese herbal medicine in order to insure miminum levels of professional competence and safety. Those who pass the acupuncture exam append the letters Dipl. Ac. (Diplomate of Acupuncture) after their names, while those who pass the Chinese herbal exam use the letters Dipl. C.H. (Diplomate of Chinese Herbs). It is our recommendation that persons wishing to experience the benefits of acupuncture and Chinese medicine should seek treatment in the U.S. only from those who are NCCA certified.

In addition, in the United States, acupuncture is a legal, independent health care profession in just slightly more than half the states. A few other states require acupuncturists to work under the supervision of M.D.s, while in a number of states, acupuncture has yet to receive legal status. In states where acupuncture is licensed and regulated, the names of acupuncture practitioners can be found in the *Yellow Pages* of your local phone book or through contacting your State Department of Health, Board of Medical Examiners, or Department of Regulatory Agencies. In states without licensure, it is doubly important to seek treatment only from NCCA diplomates.

When seeking a qualified and knowledgeable practitioner, word of mouth referrals are important. Satisfied patients are the most reliable credential a practitioner can have. It is appropriate to ask the practitioner for references from previous patients treated for the same problem. It is best to work with a practitioner who communicates effectively enough for the patient to feel understood and for the Chinese medical diagnosis and treatment plan to make sense. In all cases, a professional practitioner of Chinese medicine should be able and willing to give a written traditional Chinese diagnosis of the patient's pattern upon request.

For further information regarding the practice of Chinese medicine and acupuncture in the United States and for referrals to local professional associations and practitioners in the United States, prospective patients may contact:

98

National Commission for the Certification of Acupuncturists
P.O. Box 97075
Washington DC. 20090-7075
Tel: (202) 232-1404
Fax: (202) 462-6157

Conclusion

Pain is an unavoidable fact of human life. Research indicates most of us will experience low back pain during the course of our life. What we do to protect our back or treat our back pain is a personal choice. The current choices available for the treatment of low back pain can be confusing and overwhelming. It is hoped that this book has given you an idea of what traditional Chinese medicine has to offer you for the complete care of your low back.

Notes to Chapters

Chapter One

1 Hadler, N., "Medical Treatment of Acute Back Pain: An Overview," *Back Pain, Painful Syndromes and Muscle Spasms*, ed. by M. Jayson, R. Sweezey, J. Knoplich, A. Hubault, The Parthenon Publishing Group, 1990, p. 97

2 Waddell, G., "Understanding the Patient with Backache," *The Lumbar Spine and Back Pain*, ed. by M. Jayson, Churchill Livingstone, 1992, p. 470

3 Spangfort, E., "Disc Surgery," *Textbook of Pain*, ed. by P. Wall & R. Melzack, Churchill Livingstone, 1992, p. 795

4 Djukic, S., & Genant, H., "Magnetic Resonance Imaging," *The Lumbar Spine and Back Pain, op. cit.*, p. 263

5 Gunnar, B., "Back Schools," *The Lumbar Spine and Back Pain, op. cit.*, p. 409

6 Dobos, R., *Man Adapting*, Yale University Press, 1965, p. 323-330

7 Frymoyer, J., *New Perspectives on Back Pain*, American Academy of Orthopedic Surgeons, 1989, p. 21

8 Wall, P., "Introduction," *Textbook on Pain, op. cit.*, p. 1

9 *Ibid.*, p. 4

10 Evans, W., Jobe, W., Seibert, C., "A Cross Sectional Prevalance Study of Lumbar Degeneration in a Working Population," *Spine*, 14:60, 1989, p. 60

11 Boden, S., Davis, D., *et al.*, "Abnormal Magnetic Resonance Scans of the Lumbar Spine in Asymptomatic Subjects," *Journal of Joint and Bone Surgery*, #72A, 1990, p. 403

12 Hitseberger, W., "Abnormal Myelograms in Asymptomatic Patients," *Journal Neurosurgery*, 18:1720, 1968, p. 1722

13 Cats-Baril, W., Frymoyer, J., "The Economics of Spinal Disorders," *The*

Adult Spine, ed. by J. Frymoyer, Raven Press, 1991, p. 95

14 Mayer, T., Gatchel, R., Pollatin, P., "The Functional Restoration Programme for the Postoperative and Chronic Low Back Pain Patient," *The Lumbar Spine and Back Pain, op. cit.*, p. 517

15 Waddell, G., "Understanding the Patient with Backache," *Ibid.*, p. 469

16 Evans, W., "Education: The Primary Treatment of Low-Back Pain," *Spine Care*, ed. by A. White, Mosby, 1995, p. 347-358

Chapter Two

1 Sarno, J., *Mind Over Back Pain*, Berkely Books, 1986, p. 50

2 Jayson, M., *Back Pain, The Facts*, Oxford University Press, 1987, p. 116

Chapter Five

1 Kaptchuk, T., *The Web That Has No Weaver*, Congdon & Weed Inc., 1983, p. 164

Chapter Seven

1 Flaws, Bob, *Imperial Secrets of Health & Longevity*, Blue Poppy Press, 1994

2 Matsomoto, K., and Birch, S., *Hara Diagnosis: Reflections on the Sea*, Paradigm Publications, 1988, p. 326

3 Flaws, Bob, *Arisal of the Clear: A Simple Guide to Healthy Eating According to Traditional Chinese Medicine*, Blue Poppy Press, 1990

4 *Acute Low Back Problems in Adults: Assessment and Treatment*, No. 14, U.S. Department of Health and Human Services, Rockville, Maryland, AHCPR publication #95-0643, December, 1994, p. 1

5 *Ibid.*, p. 1

6 Hadler, N., "The Predicament of the Backache," *Journal of Occupational Medicine*, Vol. 30, #5, 1988, p. 449

7 Parry, C., "The Failed Back," *Textbook of Pain, op. cit.*, p. 341

8 Jayson, J., *op. cit.*, p. 113

9 Bain, P., Colchester, A., Nadarajah, D., "Paraplegia After Iopamidol Myelography," *The Lancet*, #27, July, 1991, p. 252

10 Malivaara, A., *et al.*, "The Treatment of Acute Low Back Pain: Bed Rest, Exercise, or Ordinary Activity?," *New England Journal of Medicine*, Vol. 332, #6, 1995, p. 351-355

11 *Acute Low Back Problems in Adults, op. cit.*, p. 13

12 *Ibid.*, p.10

13 Ronco, P., Flahault, A., "Drug-Induced End Stage Renal Disease," *New England Journal of Medicine*, Vol. 331, #25, 1994, p. 1711-1712

14 MacArthur, C., Lewis, M., Knox, E., Crawford, J., "Epidural Anaesthesia and Long Term Backache After Childbirth," *British Medical Journal*, 7 July, 1990, p. 9

15 Kabat-Zinn, J., *Full Catastrophe Living*, Delta, 1991

1
Suggested Reading & Instructional Audio and Video Tapes

Chinese Medicine

The following five books have all been written especially for the general public and capture the wide range of approaches in the practice of contemporary Chinese medicine.

The Web That Has No Weaver by Ted Kaptchuck, Congdon & Weed Inc., New York, 1983

This is the first book in English to systematically present the basic concepts of Chinese medicine. It is very readable. If one is going to read only one book on Chinese medicine, this is the one to read. It has become a classic in its own time.

Between Heaven and Earth by Harriet Beinfield & Efrem Korngold, Ballantine Books, New York, 1991

This is a more philosophical and psychological approach to Chinese medicine than *The Web*. In addition, this book is an example of how Chinese medicine is being adapted and becoming established in the West. It is also very readable. However, some of the theory is not necessarily traditionally Chinese.

The Complete Book of Chinese Health and Healing by Daniel Reid, Shambhala, Boston, 1994

This book describes the spiritual roots of Chinese medicine. Using a combination of traditional Taoist and modern biochemical language, it describes ways to protect one's health. Various *qi gong* exercises are included in this text.

Imperial Secrets of Health & Longevity by Bob Flaws, Blue Poppy Press, Boulder, CO, 1994

This book describes Chinese medicine's teachings and techniques for achieving good health and long life. Written specially for the lay reader, it covers diet, exercise, rest and relaxation, self-massage, *qi gong*, and many other aspects of achieving vibrant good health according to traditional Chinese medicine.

Arisal of the Clear: A Simple Guide to Healthy Eating According to Traditional Chinese Medicine by Bob Flaws, Blue Poppy Press, Boulder, CO, 1990

In this book, Dr. Flaws discusses in easy to understand terms the basics of Chinese dietary therapy. In particular, he emphasizes a light, easily digestible diet which promotes the production and circulation of qi and blood. He also talks about high cholesterol, food allergies, and candidiasis all from the Chinese medical point of view.

Chinese Secrets of Health & Longevity by Bob Flaws, Sounds True, Boulder, CO, 1996

This is a six tape, audio cassette "course" on Chinese health and longevity techniques for laypersons. It is loosely modeled after *Imperial Secrets* above. However, it contains more self-massage, more *qi gong* exercises, and a number of simple Chinese herbal recipes for good health. In addition, there is a whole tape devoted to the impact of emotions on health according to traditional Chinese medicine.

Western Medicine

These three books show the range of opinions in Western medicine as to the causes of low back pain.

Your Aching Back: A Doctor's Guide To Relief by August A. White M.D., Simon & Schuster/Firestone, 1990

This is a well-written book with excellent drawings of the spinal anatomy and pathology. It focuses on pathological changes of the spine as the cause of low back pain.

Back Pain: The Facts by Malcolm I.V. Jayson, M.D., Oxford University Press, New York, 1987

This book focuses on the pathological changes to structures of the low back. The author's research on pathological changes in the blood clotting system in people with certain low back problems is of special interest.

Mind Over Back Pain by John Sarno, M.D., Berkeley Books, New York, 1986

Sarno believes that the cause of low back pain is tension rather than pathological structural changes. This is a must-read book on low back pain that unites the mind and body from the Western medical point of view.

Qi Gong Books

Knocking at the Gate of Life, translated by Edward C. Chang, Ph.D., Rodale Press Inc., 1985

This book contains numerous descriptions with illustrations of healing exercises from China. It is a compilation of traditional *qi gong* and modern Chinese exercises for hundreds of physical problems including low back pain.

Ancient Way to Keep Fit compiled by Zong Wu & Li Mao, Shelter publications, 1994.

Over 30 sets of beautifully illustrated exercises taken from ancient Chinese classical works and relics.

Qi Gong Audio & Video Tapes

Blue Poppy Press distributes several instructional video and audiotapes on *qi gong*, deep relaxation, and pain relief. You may call 1-800-487-9296 to receive a complete catalog.

Qi Gong: Awakening and Mastering the Medicine Within You by Roger Jahnke, Health Action, 1995.
This video has received excellent reviews from both patients and practitioners. It is a powerful learning tool for beginners and refinement for intermediate practitioners. It has a wide array of excellent exercise forms, beautiful natural settings, and inspiring music.

Qigong: The Chinese Way of Health by Ken Cohen.
This 1 hour video has received the highest rating from *Internal Arts Magazine*. It covers the two most important basic qigong forms, healing sounds and standing meditation, which are used to cleanse the body of stagnant energy and recharge the body with fresh, healing breath.

The Way of Chi Kung by Ken Cohen, Sounds True Recordings, 1994.
This is a complete study course that teaches how to bring this natural system for mind-body healing into the lives of listeners. Covers 25 rare meditation exercises with specific instructions for breathing, postures, and imagery. 5 cassettes with vinyl binder.

Index

109

OTHER BOOKS ON CHINESE MEDICINE AVAILABLE FROM BLUE POPPY PRESS

1775 Linden Ave
Boulder, CO 80304
For ordering 1-800-487-9296
PH. 303\447-8372 FAX 303\447-0740

SEVENTY ESSENTIAL TCM FORMULAS FOR BEGINNERS by Bob Flaws, ISBN 0-936185-59-7, $19.95

CHINESE PEDIATRIC MASSAGE THERAPY: A Parent's & Practitioner's Guide to the Prevention & Treatment of Childhood Illness, by Fan Ya-li, ISBN 0-936185-54-6, $12.95

RECENT TCM RESEARCH FROM CHINA, trans. by Charles Chace & Bob Flaws, ISBN 0-936185-56-2, $18.95

EXTRA TREATISES BASED ON INVESTIGATION & INQUIRY: A Translation of Zhu Dan-xi's *Ge Zhi Yu Lun*, by Yang Shou-zhong & Duan Wu-jin, ISBN 0-936185-53-8, $15.95

A NEW AMERICAN ACUPUNCTURE by Mark Seem, ISBN 0-936185-44-9, $19.95

PATH OF PREGNANCY, VOL. I, Gestational Disorders by Bob Flaws, ISBN 0-936185-39-2, $16.95

PATH OF PREGNANCY, Vol. II, A Handbook of Traditional Chinese Postpartum Diseases

by Bob Flaws. ISBN 0-936185-42-2, $18.95

HOW TO WRITE A TCM HERBAL FORMULA A Logical Methodology for the Formulation & Administration of Chinese Herbal Medicine in Decoction, by Bob Flaws, ISBN 0-936185-49-X, $10.95

FULFILLING THE ESSENCE A Handbook of Traditional & Contemporary Treatments for Female Infertility, by Bob Flaws, ISBN 0-936185-48-1, $19.95

Li Dong-yuan's TREATISE ON THE SPLEEN & STOMACH, A Translation of the *Pi Wei Lun* by Yang Shou-zhong & Li Jian-yong, ISBN 0-936185-41-4, $21.95

SCATOLOGY & THE GATE OF LIFE: The Role of the Large Intestine in Immunity by Bob Flaws ISBN 0-936185-20-1 $14.95

MENOPAUSE A Second Spring: Making a Smooth Transition with Traditional Chinese Medicine by Honora Lee Wolfe ISBN 0-936185-18-X $14.95

How to Have A HEALTHY PREGNANCY, HEALTHY BIRTH With Traditional Chinese Medicine by Honora Lee Wolfe, ISBN 0-936185-40-6, $9.95

MIGRAINES & TRADITIONAL CHINESE MEDICINE: A Layperson's Guide by Bob Flaws ISBN 0-936185-15-5 $11.95

STICKING TO THE POINT: A Rational Methodology for the Step by Step Formulation & Administration of an Acupuncture Treatment by Bob Flaws ISBN 0-936185-17-1 $14.95

ENDOMETRIOSIS, INFERTILITY AND TRADITIONAL CHINESE MEDICINE: A Laywoman's Guide by Bob Flaws ISBN 0-936185-14-7 $9.95

THE BREAST CONNECTION: A Laywoman's Guide to the Treatment of Breast Disease by Chinese Medicine by Honora Lee Wolfe ISBN 0-936185-61-9, $9.95

NINE OUNCES: A Nine Part Program For The Prevention of AIDS in HIV Positive Persons by Bob Flaws ISBN 0-936185-12-0 $9.95

THE TREATMENT OF CANCER BY INTEGRATED CHINESE-WESTERN MEDICINE by Zhang Dai-zhao,

trans. by Zhang Ting-liang & Bob Flaws, ISBN 0-936185-11-2, $18.95

A HANDBOOK OF TRADITIONAL CHINESE DERMATOLOGY by Liang Jian-hui, trans. by Zhang Ting-liang & Bob Flaws, ISBN 0-936185-07-4 $15.95

A HANDBOOK OF TRADITIONAL CHINESE GYNECOLOGY by Zhejiang College of TCM, trans. by Zhang Ting-liang, ISBN 0-936185-06-6 (4nd edit.) $22.95

PRINCE WEN HUI'S COOK: Chinese Dietary Therapy by Bob Flaws & Honora Lee Wolfe, ISBN 0-912111-05-4, $12.95 (Published by Paradigm Press, Brookline, MA)

THE DAO OF INCREASING LONGEVITY AND CONSERVING ONE'S LIFE by Anna Lin & Bob Flaws, ISBN 0-936185-24-4 $16.95

FIRE IN THE VALLEY: The TCM Diagnosis and Treatment of Vaginal Diseases by Bob Flaws ISBN 0-936185-25-2 $16.95

HIGHLIGHTS OF ANCIENT ACUPUNCTURE PRESCRIPTIONS trans. by Honora Lee Wolfe & Rose Crescenz ISBN 0-936185-23-6 $14.95

ARISAL OF THE CLEAR: A Simple Guide to Healthy Eating According to

Traditional Chinese Medicine by Bob Flaws, ISBN #-936185-27-9 $8.95

PEDIATRIC BRONCHITIS: Its Cause, Diagnosis & Treatment According to Traditional Chinese Medicine trans. by Gao Yu-li and Bob Flaws, ISBN 0-936185-26-0 $15.95

AIDS & ITS TREATMENT ACCORDING TO TRADITIONAL CHINESE MEDICINE by Huang Bing-shan, trans. by Fu-Di & Bob Flaws, ISBN 0-936185-28-7 $24.95

ACUTE ABDOMINAL SYNDROMES: Their Diagnosis & Treatment by Combined Chinese-Western Medicine by Alon Marcus, ISBN 0-936185-31-7 $16.95

MY SISTER, THE MOON: The Diagnosis & Treatment of Menstrual Diseases by Traditional Chinese Medicine by Bob Flaws, ISBN 0-936185-34-1, $24.95

FU QING-ZHU'S GYNECOLOGY trans. by Yang Shou-zhong and Liu Da-wei, ISBN 0-936185-35-X, $22.95

FLESHING OUT THE BONES: The Importance of Case Histories in Chinese Medicine trans. by Charles Chace. ISBN 0-936185-30-9, $18.95

CLASSICAL MOXIBUSTION SKILLS in Contemporary Clinical Practice by Sung Baek, ISBN 0-936185-16-3 $12.95

THE MEDICAL I CHING: Oracle of the Healer Within by Miki Shima, OMD, ISBN 0-936185-38-4, $19.95

MASTER TONG'S ACUPUNCTURE: An Ancient Lineage for Modern Practice, trans. and commentary by Miriam Lee, OMD, ISBN 0-936185-37-6, $19.95

A HANDBOOK OF TCM UROLOGY & MALE SEXUAL DYSFUNCTION by Anna Lin, OMD, ISBN 0-936185-36-8, $16.95

PMS: Its Cause, Diagnosis & Treatment According to Traditional Chinese Medicine by Bob Flaws ISBN 0-936185-22-8 $14.95

MASTER HUA'S CLASSIC OF THE CENTRAL VISCERA by Hua Tuo, ISBN 0-936185-43-0, $21.95

THE HEART & ESSENCE OF DAN-XI'S METHODS OF TREATMENT by Xu Dan-xi, trans. by Yang Shou-zhong, ISBN 0-926185-49-X, $21.95

STATEMENTS OF FACT IN TRADITIONAL CHINESE MEDICINE by Bob Flaws, ISBN 0-936185-52-X, $10.95

IMPERIAL SECRETS OF
HEALTH & LONGEVITY by
Bob Flaws, ISBN 0-936185-51-1,
$9.95

THE SYSTEMATIC CLASSIC
OF ACUPUNCTURE &
MOXIBUSTION (Jia Yi Jing) by
Huang-fu Mi, trans. by Yang
Shou-zhong and Charles Chace,
ISBN 0-936185-29-5, $79.95

CHINESE MEDICINAL WINES
& ELIXIRS by Bob Flaws, ISBN 0-
936185-58-9, $18.95

THE DIVINELY
RESPONDING CLASSIC: A
Translation of the Shen Ying Jing
from the Zhen Jiu Da Cheng,
trans. by Yang Shou-zhong and
Liu Feng-ting ISBN 0-936185-55-
4

PAO ZHI: An Introduction to
Processing Chinese Medicinals to
Enhance Their Therapeutic
Effect, by Philippe Sionneau,
ISBN 0-936185-62-1, $34.95

THE BOOK OF JOOK: Chinese
Medicinal Porridges, An
Alternative to the Typical
Western Breakfast, by Bob Flaws,
ISBN0-936185-60-0, $16.95

SHAOLIN SECRET
FORMULAS for the Treatment
of External Injuries, by De Chan,
ISBN 0-936185-08-2, $18.95

AGING & BLOOD STASIS: A
New Approach to TCM
Geriatrics, by Yan De-xin, ISBN
0-936185-63-5, $21.95

CHINESE MEDICAL
PALMISTRY: Your Health in
Your Hand, by Zong Xiao-fan &
Gary Liscum, ISBN 0-936185-64-
3, $15.95

THE SECRET OF CHINESE
PULSE DIAGNOSIS by Bob
Flaws, ISBN 0-936185-67-8,
$17.95.

LOW BACK PAIN: Care &
Prevention with Traditional
Chinese Medicine by Douglas
Frank, ISBN 0-936185-66-X,
$9.95